Praise for *The G.I. Diet* by Rick Gallop

"Dieting has never been made easier and more satisfying."
—Lucy Waverman, author and food columnist, *Globe & Mail*

"An innovative, realistic, uncomplicated long-term approach to successful weight management."
—Dr. Michael Sole, M.D.;
Fellow of the American College of Cardiology

"If you can understand a stoplight, you can lose weight on this amazing diet."
—Marilyn Linton, health columnist, *Toronto Sun*

"Excellent . . . This book is timely, of tremendous relevance, easy to read, practical and explodes several myths."
—Dr. Sudi Devanesen, M.D.;
Canadian College of Family Physicians

"This is my diet book forever."
—Barbara Amiel Black, columnist for the
Chicago Sun Times and *London Daily Telegraph*

"An excellent guide for people looking to reduce their risk of cardiovascular disease."
—Dr. David Jenkins, M.D., Ph.D., D.Sc.;
Professor, Department of Nutritional Sciences,
Faculty of Medicine, University of Toronto

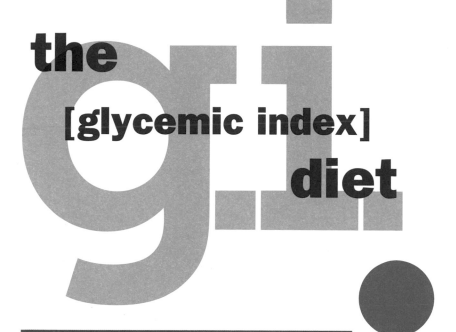

the g.i. [glycemic index] diet

THE EASY, HEALTHY WAY TO Permanent Weight Loss

RICK GALLOP

FOREWORD BY EDMUND H. SONNENBLICK, M.D.

workman publishing ▪ new york

First published in somewhat different form by
Random House Canada.
This U.S. edition published by arrangement with
Random House Canada, a division of Random House
of Canada Limited.

Library of Congress Cataloging-in-Publication Data
available upon request.

ISBN 0-7611-3178-7

Cover design by Paul Gamarello
Interior design by Barbara Balch

Workman books are available at special discounts when
purchased in bulk for premiums and sales promotions as
well as for fund-raising or educational use. Special
editions or book excerpts can be created to specification.
For details, contact the Special Sales Director at the
address below.

Workman Publishing Company, Inc.
708 Broadway
New York, NY 10003-9555

www.workman.com

Printed in November 2003

10 9 8 7 6 5 4

Acknowledgments

While I was writing *The G.I. Diet*, I was also running the Heart and Stroke Foundation of Ontario, which has thirty-six offices and forty-five thousand volunteers and raises more than $100 million annually. The book was an enormous drain on my family time, and my wife, Ruth, bore the brunt of my preoccupation. Despite this, she was my cheerleader, culinary adviser, and coach. Without her encouragement and support, I doubt that I would have ever completed this book.

Dr. Michael Sole, cardiologist and researcher, provided invaluable advice and counsel. I am also deeply indebted to Dr. Ed Sonnenblick, one of the most eminent cardiologists in the United States, for believing in the value of the G.I. Diet and writing the foreword to the book.

Among the many sources of information on the glycemic index, the most authoritative voice is Professor Jennie Brand-Miller at the University of Sydney. Her pioneering work in this field has been truly outstanding.

Maureen Dwight, my physiotherapist, who solved my lower-back problem with an exercise program that is now a regular part of my life, was invaluable in helping put together the exercise chapter and appendix. Maureen is the director of the Orthopaedic Therapy Clinic in Toronto.

My thanks to my friends at Random House of Canada and Workman Publishing in New York: Anne Collins for encouraging me to write the book and Stacey Cameron, Suzanne Rafer, and Beth Doty for keeping me on track with wonderful editing and direction.

Finally, I must thank all my friends and associates who took part in my dietary research. Their feedback provided the focus and essence of the G.I. Diet.

Contents

Foreword by Edmund H. Sonnenblick, M.D. ix

Introduction xi

chapter one | The Problem 2

chapter two | How Much Weight Should I Lose? 16

chapter three | Phase I 25

chapter four | Ready, Set, Go! 58

chapter five | The Green-Light Glossary 64

chapter six | Meal Ideas 70

chapter seven | Phase II 96

chapter eight | Exercise 104

chapter nine | Health 117

chapter ten | Supplements 121

Appendixes

I: The Complete G.I. Diet Food Guide 125

II: Green-Light Kitchen Cupboard Essentials 133

III: G.I. Diet Shopping List 135

IV: Dining Out and Travel Tips 137

V: Exercise Calorie Counter 139

VI: Strengthening & Resistance Exercises 143

VII: The Ten Golden G.I. Diet Rules 151

Index 154

Foreword

Excess weight and obesity, with their co-morbid consequences such as hypertension, stroke, diabetes, and atherosclerotic vascular disease, are the plagues of an adequately fed society. Rick Gallop has now put together an approach to the problem that provides not only a way to lose unnecessary weight, but a way to keep from regaining it. He has formulated the Glycemic Index (G.I.) Diet, which expertly explains what causes us to gain weight, how to lose it, and how to keep it off. It not only makes sense, it works, bringing together sound science and a very practical approach. He tells us what to eat and why. He also tells us what not to eat and why. Moreover, this approach avoids hunger and still provides satisfaction.

Losing weight is relatively easy with many "fad" diets; maintaining the loss with these diets is difficult and largely impossible to sustain. Rick Gallop has found the key to permanent weight loss and he's here to tell us how. Avoiding obesity and staying that way not only makes us look and feel better, but helps us to control high blood pressure and to prevent the development of diabetes, thus reducing the risk of heart disease, vascular disease, and stroke.

The G.I. Diet has already been an immense success in the hands of thousands of Canadian and British readers, and so should this new American edition.

—Edmund H. Sonnenblick, M.D.

Edmond J. Safra Professor of Medicine and former Chief of Cardiology at the Albert Einstein College of Medicine, New York City, New York

Introduction

During the fifteen years that I was president of the Heart and Stroke Foundation of Ontario, my job was to raise funds for research into heart disease and stroke and to promote healthy lifestyle choices among Canadians to reduce their risk for those diseases. The foundation, a sister organization to the American Heart Association, has developed the most comprehensive set of heart disease, stroke, and healthy lifestyle resources in Canada. We now know that smoking, high blood pressure, high blood cholesterol, a sedentary lifestyle, and being overweight are all major risk factors for heart attacks and strokes. So a few years ago, when I was twenty pounds overweight, I knew I had to reduce. And with all the information and resources I had, I thought I knew how: I went out and bought a Nordic ski machine and a stationary bike, and I started working out every day. But no matter how hard I exercised, I found I could only stabilize, not lose, the weight. For the first time in my life, I realized I had to go on a diet.

Conventional nutritional wisdom at the time recommended a low-fat, high-carbohydrate diet. All I had to do was to stop eating fatty foods like cheese and ice cream, and to start eating more low-fat carbohydrates like pasta, rice, and vegetables—right? Wrong. Though I stuck diligently to the diet, eating pasta and tomato sauce instead of steak and Caesar salad, I wasn't losing any weight at all. In frustration, I turned to the filing cabinets at the Heart and Stroke Foundation of Ontario. The foundation receives literally hundreds of diet books, products, and recipes every year, all hoping for support or endorsement. Looking through the files, I quickly ruled out food-specific diets, such as the grapefruit and banana diets, because they have no scientific basis, are risky to your health, and are impossible to sustain over the long term.

I also decided to avoid high-protein diets, since various studies had found them to be a real health hazard. The fact that the high-protein, low-carbohydrate diet that was very popular in the 1970s is back in the headlines again as the weight-loss choice of the stars is alarming news. This diet, popularized by Dr. Robert C. Atkins, is potentially a serious long-term risk to health.

The diet is based on high intake of animal protein and saturated fat with minimal carbohydrates. It works by the body burning fat for energy instead of carbohydrates. While that sounds like a good idea in principle, the process called ketosis has the potential to create a dangerous electrolyte imbalance and an acid buildup in the blood that can cause kidney damage, kidney stones, and osteoporosis by leaching the calcium from bones. Side effects include fatigue, headache, nausea, faintness, and bad breath. In addition, the high levels of red meat and saturated fat in this diet increase the risk of heart disease, stroke, and some cancers.

But what is especially important is what the high-protein, high-saturated-fat diet doesn't contain. By minimizing carbohydrates, it severely limits one of the three food groups that virtually every health authority agrees are essential for good health. Such a drastic reduction in fruits, vegetables, whole grains, and legumes deprives the body of essential minerals, vitamins, and fiber. These carbohydrates are critical for a healthy body and for reducing the risk of heart disease, stroke, and colorectal and prostate cancer.

While there is clear evidence that this high-protein diet enables you to lose weight in the short term, the rate of long-term weight loss is not markedly different from other major recognized diets. In addition, a large degree of the weight loss is due to the diuretic nature of this diet. This means it's the loss of water—not fat—that accounts for much of the weight loss. People coming off high-protein diets usually put on weight rapidly as the water levels in their tissues return to normal.

So, diets based on a single food and high-protein diets were out. I was still left with a whole host of diets to try, and I selected one that appeared to be based on sound nutritional principles. After several unsuccessful months with that one, I embarked on another, and then a few months later, another. I don't know how many of them I tried. I counted calories. I studied labels—a real challenge trying to make sense of servings, fat grams, and daily percentages. I starved. I hallucinated about food. Sometimes I did lose a few pounds, but then I'd hit the inevitable plateau, unable to go any further. And since I was constantly hungry, I'd soon start eating what I wanted and gain back the few pounds I'd managed to lose.

The Answer: The Glycemic Index

It seemed as if I was destined to spend the rest of my life overweight. It was the most discouraging thing I have ever experienced. I couldn't understand why losing weight was so difficult, and I felt there had to be a way to slim down and maintain a healthy weight without having to feel hungry every moment of the day, jeopardizing my health, or requiring a Ph.D. in math to calculate various formulas and ratios. I was determined to find a diet that would work not only for myself, but also for others in the same boat.

My quest eventually led me to one of the nutritional researchers supported by the Heart and Stroke Foundation of Ontario. He introduced me to the G.I., or Glycemic Index, through a book called *The Zone* by Dr. Barry Sears. The Zone Diet is based on the principles of the G.I., which measures the speed at which your body breaks down carbohydrates and converts them to glucose, the primary fuel your body uses for energy. The faster the food breaks down, the higher the rating on the index. When trying to lose weight, it is critical to avoid foods that have a high G.I. and to eat low-G.I. foods instead. The Glycemic Index was invented by Dr. David Jenkins, a professor of nutrition at the University of Toronto. Since he was living in my hometown, I decided to pay him a visit.

A lean Englishman who clearly practices what he preaches, Dr. Jenkins explained that early in his research career he became interested in diabetes, a disease that hampers the body's ability to process glucose. Glucose therefore stays in the bloodstream instead of going into the cells, resulting in hyperglycemia and potentially coma. At the time Dr. Jenkins was beginning his research, carbohydrates were severely restricted in a diabetic's diet, as they quickly boost the glucose level in the bloodstream. But because the primary role of carbohydrates is to provide the body with energy, diabetics were having to make up the lack of calories through a high-fat diet, which does not boost glucose levels. As a result, many diabetics were increasingly at risk of heart disease, since fat is a critical factor in the development of that disease. Doctors were in a real quandary: although they were saving diabetics from starvation, they were accelerating their patients' risk of heart disease.

Dr. Jenkins wondered if all carbohydrates are the same. Are some digested more quickly and as a result raise blood glucose levels faster than others? And are others "slow-release," resulting in only a marginal increase in blood glucose? The answer, Jenkins discovered, is yes. He published an index—the Glycemic Index—in 1980, showing the various rates at which carbohydrates break down and release glucose into the bloodstream.

The Key to Permanent Weight Loss

I decided to try The Zone Diet. To my amazement and delight, I lost the twenty pounds that had been plaguing me for so long. I invited some of my friends and associates to try it as well. By the end of twelve months, however, 95 percent had dropped out. They cited two principal reasons for their inability to stick to the diet: (1) It was too complex for everyday life, requiring them to count grams and calculate formulas and ratios; and (2) They were always feeling hungry or deprived, which is the death knell for any diet.

The 5 percent who managed to hang in were so happy with their success that I received numerous e-mails from them describing how important their weight control was in their lives. Here are a few of their comments:

"Overall, I have lost twenty-two pounds. And I feel more ener-gized. . . . I don't even notice that I'm eating differently. I certainly don't feel like I'm on a diet. I just feel like I eat in a new way."

"Well, with Thanksgiving, two large family dinners, weekend guests, lunches with friends, being on the road, and my love of wine and food, I have managed to lose fifteen pounds. I can honestly say my energy is better—I'm not falling asleep in front of the TV anymore."

Dismayed by the 95 percent dropout rate but bolstered by the successful 5 percent, I set out to address the two key impediments to success: complexity and hunger. The result is this book. The G.I. Diet is simple to follow and will not leave you feeling hungry. The plan comprises a unique combination of foods that have two essential characteristics: They make you feel full for a longer time, so you are naturally inclined to eat less, and they are low-calorie. If you, like me, have been reading other recent diet books, you will have noticed that the word *calorie* is rarely used. But lowering caloric intake is the only route to weight loss, and all those diets are, in fact, low-calorie; it's just that the word has been omitted. With The G.I. Diet, you won't need to count calories, or weigh or meas-ure your food. I've done all the math for you to create the easiest eating plan possible, one that reflects the demands of the busy world we live in. While most diet books take three hundred pages or more to make their point, *The G.I. Diet* is simple and concise, with little scientific jargon. Its most important feature is that *it works.* You'll find it so simple to follow, so effective, you'll never have to pick up a diet book again.

Please visit my Web site at **www.gidiet.com**
for the latest developments in nutrition and health.

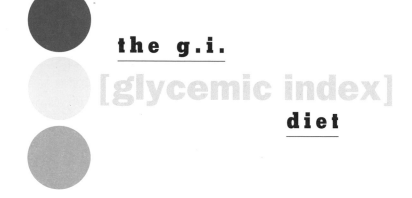

the g.i.

[glycemic index]

diet

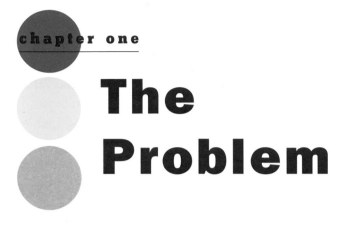

chapter one

The
Problem

While I was waging my personal battle of the bulge, I couldn't help but be struck by the number of people who were engaged in the same struggle. The statistics are truly astonishing: 61 percent of Americans are overweight and an incredible one in four—double the rate of twenty years ago—is obese. The United States unfortunately leads the international stage in the heavyweight stakes. Here are some recent comparisons with other major Western countries:

	% overweight	% obese
U.S.	61	24
U.K.	58	19
Australia	57	18
Canada	48	15
France	40	15
Sweden	40	11
Italy	34	10
Germany	27	18

Sources: British Heart Foundation, World Health Organization, and International Obesity Task Force

What's happened to us? Why have we gained so much weight in the past twenty years?

The simple explanation is that people are eating too many calories. Unless one denies the basic laws of thermodynamics, the equation never changes: Consume more calories than you expend and the surplus is stored in the body as fat. That's the inescapable fact. But that doesn't explain why people today are eating more calories than they used to. To answer that question, we must first understand the three key components of any diet—fats, carbohydrates, and proteins—and how they function in our digestive system. Since fats are probably the least well understood, let's start with them.

FATS

Fat is definitely a bad word these days, and it engenders an enormous amount of confusion and contradiction. But are you aware that fats are absolutely essential to your diet? They contain various key elements that are crucial to the digestive process.

The next fact might also surprise you: Fat does not necessarily make you fat. The quantity you consume does. And that's something that's often difficult to control, because your body *loves* fat. Nonfat foods require lots of processing to be transformed into those fat cells around your waist and hips; fatty foods just slide right in. Processing takes energy, and your body hates wasting energy. It needs to expend about 20 to 25 percent of the energy it gets from a nonfat food just to process it. So your body definitely prefers fat, and as we all know from personal experience, it will do everything it can to persuade you to eat more of it. That's why fatty foods like juicy steaks, chocolate cake, and decadent ice cream taste so good to us. But because fat contains twice as many calories per gram as carbohydrates and proteins, we really have to be careful about the amount of fat we eat.

In addition to limiting *how much* fat we consume, we must also pay attention to the *type* of fat. While the type of fat has no effect on our weight, it is critical to our health—especially our heart health.

There are four types of fat: the best, the good, the bad, and the really ugly.

The "really ugly" fats are potentially the most dangerous. They are vegetable oils that have been heat-treated to make them thicken. These hydrogenated oils, or trans fatty acids, take on the worst characteristics of saturated fats (see below), so don't use them, and avoid snack foods, baked goods, and cereals that contain them. Check the label for "hydrogenated oils" or "partially hydrogenated oils."

The "bad" fats are called saturated fats, and they are easily recognizable because they almost always come from animal sources and they solidify at room temperature. Butter, cheese, hard (stick) margarine, and meat are all high in saturated fats. There are a couple of others you should be aware of, too. Coconut oil and palm oil are two vegetable oils that are saturated, and because they are cheap, they are used in many snack foods, especially cookies. Saturated fats are a principal cause of heart disease because they boost cholesterol, which in turn thickens arteries and causes heart attack and stroke.

Fifteen or so years ago, a wealthy American industrialist had a heart attack. Like many successful businessmen, he hated surprises, and he wanted to know what had caused the unexpected turn in his health. When he discovered that many leading food products contain tropical oils such as palm and coconut, he took out a full-page ad in *The Wall Street Journal* with the headline "These Nine Products Are Killing Americans." Within forty-eight hours, eight of the nine products were reformulated without the tropical oils. Check your labels.

The "good" fats are called polyunsaturated fats, and they are cholesterol-free. Most vegetable oils, such as corn and sunflower, fall into this category.

What you should really be eating, however, are monounsaturated fats, the "best," which are found in olives, peanuts, almonds, and olive and canola oils. Monounsaturated fats have a beneficial effect on cholesterol and are good for your heart. (See chapter 9 for more information on cholesterol and heart disease.) Though fancy olive oils are expensive, you can get the same health benefits from reasonably priced house brands at your supermarket. Olive oil is used extensively in the famed Mediterranean diet, which is also rich in fruits and vegetables. Because of their diet, southern Europeans have some of the lowest rates of heart disease in the world, and obesity is not a problem in those countries. So look for monounsaturated fats and oils on food labels.

Another highly beneficial oil, which is in a category of its own, contains a wonderful ingredient called omega-3—found in deep-sea fish such as salmon and in flaxseed and canola oils. It's extremely good for your heart health (see page 123).

So we know that it's important to avoid the bad and the really ugly fats and to incorporate the best fats into our diets to make our hearts healthy. Many of us have tried to lower our fat intake by using leaner cuts of meat and drinking lower-fat milk. But even with these modifications, our fat consumption hasn't decreased. Why? Because many of our favorite foods—such as crackers,

COOKING OILS/FATS

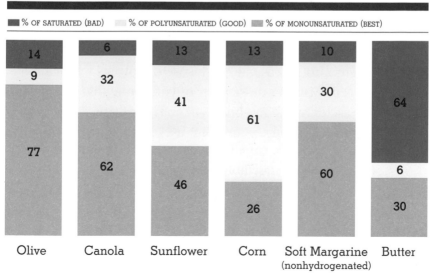

■ % OF SATURATED (BAD)   % OF POLYUNSATURATED (GOOD)   ■ % OF MONOUNSATURATED (BEST)

Olive	Canola	Sunflower	Corn	Soft Margarine (nonhydrogenated)	Butter
14	6	13	13	10	
9	32	41	61	30	64
77	62	46	26	60	6
					30

muffins, cereals, and fast foods—contain hidden fats. Detecting them often seems to require an advanced degree in nutrition, even with the labeling of nutritional components on food packaging.

So we're not eating less fat, but, contrary to popular belief, neither are we eating more. Fat consumption in this country has remained virtually constant over the past ten years, while over-weight numbers have doubled. Obviously, fat isn't the culprit. What has increased is our consumption of grain. Grain is a carbo-hydrate, so let's look at how carbohydrates work.

---

to sum up

1. Eat less fat overall and look for low-fat alternatives to your current diet.

2. Eat the monounsaturated and polyunsaturated fats only.

CARBOHYDRATES

Carbohydrates are the primary source of energy for your body. They are found in grains, vegetables, fruits, legumes, and dairy products. Your body takes in carbohydrates from these foods and converts them into glucose. The glucose dissolves in your blood-stream and is diverted to those parts of your body that use energy, like your muscles and your brain. (It may surprise you to know that when you are resting, your brain uses about two thirds of the glucose in your system!)

Carbohydrates, obviously, are essential for your body to func-tion. They are rich in fiber, vitamins, and minerals, including anti-oxidants, which we now believe play a critical role in protecting against disease, especially heart disease and cancer. For years we've been advised by doctors, nutritionists, and the government to eat a low-fat, high-carbohydrate diet—just look at the USDA Food Pyramid (see page 28), where grains form the base. The trouble with this is that it has encouraged us all to rely too much on grain-based products. Just look at the amount of space dedicated to them in our supermarkets today: huge cracker, cookie, and snack-food sections; whole aisles of cereals; numerous shelves of pastas and noodles; and baskets and baskets of bagels, rolls, muffins, and loaves of bread. I can remember when bagels were exclusive to the Jewish community; now most food stores carry half a dozen different varieties, and chains of bagel stores are spread across the country. Muffins were never as abundant as they are today.

Another modern food sensation has been pasta, once viewed as an ethnic specialty in the United States and Canada. That's hard to believe today, with pasta as a staple on most restaurant menus and every family's shopping list. U.S. pasta consumption has nearly doubled over the past ten years or so. And our snack-food options have multiplied: crackers, tortilla chips, corn chips, pretzels, and countless varieties of cookies, to name just a few.

In 1970, the average American and Canadian ate about 135 pounds of grain per year. By 2000, that figure had risen to *200* pounds. That's a nearly 50 percent increase! But why should we be concerned about this? Aren't wheat, corn, and rice low-fat? How could grain be making us fat?

The answer lies in the *type* of grain we're eating today, most of which is in the form of white flour. White flour starts off as whole wheat. At the mill, the whole wheat is steamed and scarified by tiny razor-sharp blades to remove the bran, or outer shell, and the endosperm, the next layer. Then the wheat germ and oil are removed because they turn rancid too quickly to be considered commercially viable. What's left after all that processing is unbleached flour, which is then whitened and used to make almost all the breads, bagels, muffins, cookies, crackers, cereals, and pastas we consume. Even many "brown" breads are simply artificially colored white bread.

It's not just grain that's highly processed nowadays. A hundred

GRAIN CONSUMPTION (POUNDS PER CAPITA)

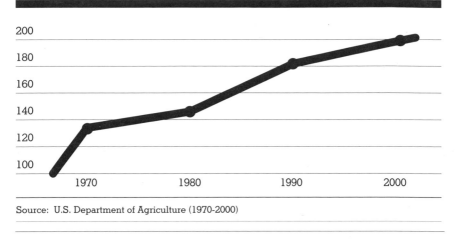

Source: U.S. Department of Agriculture (1970-2000)

years ago, most of the food people ate came straight from the farm to the dinner table. Lack of refrigeration and scant knowledge of food chemistry meant that most food remained in its original state. However, advances in science, along with the migration of many women out of the kitchen and into the workforce, led to a revolution in prepared foods. Everything became geared to speed and simplicity of preparation. Today's high-speed flour mills use steel rollers rather than the traditional grinding stones to produce an extraordinarily fine-ground product, ideal for producing light and fluffy breads and pastries. We now have instant rice and potatoes, as well as entire meals that are ready to eat after just a few minutes in the microwave.

The trouble with all this is that the more a food is processed beyond its natural state, the less processing your body has to do to digest it. And the quicker you digest your food, the sooner you are hungry again, and the more you tend to eat. We all know the difference between eating a bowl of old-fashioned slow-cooking oatmeal and a bowl of sugary cold cereal. The oatmeal stays with you—it "sticks to your ribs," as my mother used to say—whereas you are looking for your next meal an hour after eating the bowl of sugary cereal. That's why our ancestors did not have the obesity problem we have today; their foods were basically unprocessed and natural. All of the great food companies, such as Kraft, General Foods, Kellogg's, McCain, Nabisco, and Del Monte, only started processing and packaging natural foods in the past century.

Our fundamental problem, then, is that we are eating foods that are too easily digested by our bodies. Clearly, we can't wind back the clock to simpler times, but we need somehow to slow down the digestive process so we feel hungry less often. How can we do that? Well, we have to eat foods that are "slow-release," that break down at a slow and steady rate in our digestive system, leaving us feeling fuller for longer.

How do we identify those "slow-release" foods? There are two clues. The first is the amount of fiber in the food. Fiber, in simple terms, provides low-calorie filler. It does double duty, in fact: It literally fills up your stomach, so you feel satiated, and your body takes much longer to break it down, so it stays with you longer and slows down the digestive process. There are two forms of fiber: soluble and insoluble. Soluble fiber is found in foods like oatmeal, beans, barley, and citrus fruits, and has been shown to lower blood cholesterol levels. Insoluble fiber is important for normal bowel function and is typically found in whole wheat breads and cereals and most vegetables.

The second tool in identifying slow-release foods is the Glycemic Index, which I will now explain. It is the core of this diet and the key to successful weight management.

to sum up

Eat foods that have not been highly processed and that do not contain highly processed ingredients.

THE GLYCEMIC INDEX

The Glycemic Index measures the speed at which you digest food and convert it to glucose, your body's energy source. The faster the food breaks down, the higher the rating on the index. The index sets glucose at 100 and scores all foods against that number. Here are some examples:

GLYCEMIC INDEX RATINGS

glucose(sugar) =100

Baguette	95	Orange	44
Rice (instant)	87	All-Bran	43
Cornflakes	84	Oatmeal	42
Potato (baked)	84	Peach	42
Doughnut	76	Spaghetti	41
Cheerios	75	Tomato	38
Bagel	72	Apple	38
Raisins	64	Yogurt (low-fat)	33
Rice (basmati)	58	Fettuccine	32
Muffin (bran)	56	Beans	31
Potato (new/boiled)	56	Grapefruit	25
Popcorn (microwave light)	55	Yogurt (nonfat/no sugar)	14

The chart on the next page illustrates the impact of sugar on the level of glucose in your bloodstream compared with kidney beans, which have a low G.I. rating. As you can see, there is a dramatic difference between the two. Sugar is quickly converted into glucose, which dissolves in your bloodstream, spiking the blood's glucose level. Sugars also disappear quickly, leaving you wanting more. Have you ever eaten a large Chinese meal, with lots of noodles and rice, only to find yourself hungry again an hour or two later? That's because your body rapidly converted the rice and noodles, both high-G.I. foods, to glucose, which then quickly disappeared from your bloodstream. Something most of us experience regularly is the lethargy that follows an hour or so after a fast-food lunch, which generally consists of high-G.I. foods. The surge of glucose followed by the rapid drain leaves us starved of energy. So what do we do? Around mid-afternoon, we look for a quick sugar fix, or snack, to bring us out of the slump. A few cookies or a bag of chips cause another rush of glucose, which disappears a short time later—and so the vicious cycle continues. No wonder we're a nation of snackers!

When you eat a high-G.I. food and experience a rapid spike in blood sugar, your pancreas releases the hormone insulin. Insulin does two things extremely well. First, it reduces the level of glucose in your bloodstream by diverting it into various body tissues for immediate short-term use or by storing it as fat—which is why glucose disappears so quickly. Second, it inhibits the conversion of body fat back into glucose for the body to burn. This evolutionary feature is a throwback to the days when our ancestors were hunter-gatherers, habitually experiencing times of feast or famine. When food was in abundance, the body stored its surplus as fat to tide it over during the inevitable days of famine. Insulin was the champion in this process, both helping to accumulate fat and then guarding its depletion.

G.I. IMPACT ON SUGAR LEVELS

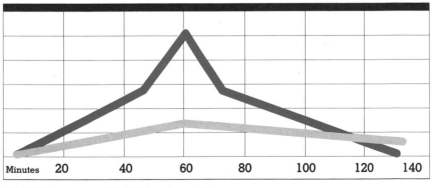

| Minutes | 20 | 40 | 60 | 80 | 100 | 120 | 140 |

G.I. 100 Glucose ■■   G.I. 27 Kidney Beans ▨

Today, everything has changed except our stomachs. A digestive system that has taken millions of years to evolve is, in a comparative blink of an eye, expected to cope with a food revolution. We don't have to hunt for food anymore; we have a guaranteed supply of highly processed foods with a multitude of tempting flavors and textures at the supermarket. Not only are we consuming more easily digested calories, but we're not expending as much energy in finding our food and keeping ourselves warm—the two major preoccupations of our ancestors.

The production of insulin is triggered by the presence of glucose in the bloodstream. Since its two primary roles are to store that glucose as fat and to act as sentry to keep those fat cells intact, it is crucial to maintain low insulin levels when you are trying to lose weight, and that means avoiding high-G.I. foods. Low-G.I. foods such as apples are like the tortoise to the high-G.I. foods' hare. They break down in your digestive system at a slow, steady rate. You don't get a quick sugar fix when you eat them, but, tortoiselike, they stay the course, so that you feel full longer. So if you want to lose weight, you must stick to low-G.I. foods.

But the fact that a food has a low G.I. rating does not necessarily make it desirable. The other critical factor determining whether a food will allow you to lose weight is its calorie content. It's the combination of low-G.I. foods with few calories—that is, low in sugar and fat—that is the "magic bullet" of the G.I. Diet. Low-G.I., low-calorie foods make you feel more satiated than do foods with a high G.I. and calorie level. Later in this book, I will provide a comprehensive chart identifying the foods that will make you fat and those that will allow you to lose weight. Don't expect all the low-G.I. foods to be tasteless and boring! There are many delicious and satisfying choices that will make you feel as though you aren't even on a diet.

I've already mentioned two of the principal factors that contribute to a food's G.I. rating: The degree of processing it undergoes before it is digested and how much fiber it contains.

But there are two other important components that inhibit the rapid breakdown of food in our digestive system, and they are fat and protein. The influence of these two factors can lead to some surprising, and confusing, results. Peanut butter, for example, has a low G.I. because of its high fat and protein content. Similarly, whole milk has a lower G.I. than skim, and fruitcake has a lower G.I. than melba toast. Fat, like fiber, acts as a brake in the digestive process. When combined with other foods, it becomes a barrier to digestive juices. It also signals the brain that you are satisfied and do not require more food. However, these low-G.I., high-fat foods are calorie-dense, with twice the number of calories per gram that carbohydrates and protein have, and they're not compatible with this diet plan. Plus, we know that many fats are harmful to your heart. Since protein also acts as a brake in the digestive process, let's look at it in more detail.

---

to sum up

1. Low-G.I. foods are slower to digest, so you feel satiated longer.

2. Keeping insulin levels low inhibits the formation of fat and assists in the conversion of fat back into energy.

3. The key to losing weight is to eat low-G.I., low-calorie foods.

PROTEIN

As with fat, there's been a great deal of misinformation and nonsense about protein and its role in our diet. For a long time, nutritionists and dietitians didn't think protein was a factor in weight control. Then, in the 1970s, high-protein diets became all the rage. They promoted the consumption of all the protein and fat you could eat while minimizing carbohydrates. This type of diet has become all the rage once again, but as we now know, it's harmful to your long-term health. High-protein diets have rightly been criticized by nutritionists and doctors alike.

Let's get the facts about protein straight. Proteins are an essential part of your diet. One half of your dry body weight is made up of protein, including your muscles, organs, skin, and hair. Protein is required to build and repair body tissue, and it figures in nearly all metabolic reactions.

Protein is also much more effective than carbohydrates or fat in satisfying hunger. It will make you feel fuller longer, which is why you should always try to incorporate some protein in every meal and snack. It will help keep you alert and feeling full. Again, however, the type of protein you consume is important. Proteins are found in a broad range of food products, both animal and vegetable, and not just in red meat and whole dairy products, which are high in saturated, or "bad," fat.

So what sort of protein should you include in your diet? Choose low-fat proteins: lean or low-fat meats that have been trimmed of any visible fat; skinless poultry; fresh, frozen, or canned seafood (but not the kind that's coated with batter, which is invariably high in fat); low-fat dairy products such as skim milk (believe it or not, after a couple of weeks of drinking it, it tastes just like 2%); low-fat yogurt (look for the artificially sweetened versions, as many manufacturers pump up the sugar as they drop the fat) and low-fat cottage cheese; low-fat and low-cholesterol liquid eggs; tofu; and soy or whey protein powder, which is great for sprinkling on meals. To most people's surprise, the best source of protein may well be the humble bean. Beans are high-protein, low-fat, and high-fiber, and they break down slowly in your digestive system, so you feel fuller longer. They can also be added to foods like soups and salads to boost their protein and fiber content. Nuts, too, are a fine source of protein, with a good monounsaturated fat content. However, because they are so high in fat, you must limit the quantity.

One of the most important things about protein is to spread your daily allowance across all your meals. Too often we grab a hasty breakfast of coffee and toast—a protein-free meal. Lunch is sometimes not much better: a bowl of hot vegetable soup or a green salad with a roll and butter. Where's the protein? A typical afternoon snack of a cookie, a piece of fruit, or chips contains not a gram of protein. Generally, it's not until dinner that we include protein in our meal, usually our entire daily recommended allowance plus some extra. Because protein is a critical brain food, providing amino acids for the neurotransmitters that relay messages in the brain, it would be better to load up on protein earlier in the day rather than later. That would give you an alert and active mind for your daily activities. However, as I have said, the best solution is to spread your protein consumption throughout the day. This will help keep you on the ball and feeling full.

Now that we know how fats, carbohydrates, and proteins work in our digestive system and what makes us gain weight, let's use the science to put together an eating plan that will take off the extra pounds. First, let's look at how much weight you should be trying to lose.

---

to sum up

1. Include some protein in all your meals and snacks.
2. Eat only low-fat protein, preferably from both animal and vegetable sources.

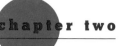

chapter two

How Much Weight Should I Lose?

I n this age of excessively and often unhealthily skinny super-
models and TV stars, it's easy to lose sight of what is a healthy
weight. Your skin, bones, organs, hair—everything—contribute to
your total weight. The only part that you want to reduce is your
excess fat, so that's what we have to determine.

There have been many techniques designed to measure excess
fat, from measuring pinches of fat (which can be quite misleading)
to convoluted formulas and tables requiring higher math. The
traditional method, relating weight directly to height through the
Metropolitan Life tables, does not tell you how much body fat
you're carrying around your waist, hips, and thighs, and that's the
information you really need to know. So the best method is the
Body Mass Index, or BMI. I've included a BMI table on pages
18–19, and it's very simple to use. Just find your height in the left
vertical column and go across the table until you reach your
weight. At the top of that column is your BMI, which is an accu-
rate estimate of the amount of body fat you're carrying.

BMI values less than 19 are considered underweight, while those between 25 and 30 are classified as overweight. BMI values over 30 are classified as obese. However, if you are under 5 feet, are elderly, or are overly muscled (and you really have to be a dedicated bodybuilder to qualify), these numbers in all probability do not apply to you.

The ideal BMI is between 19 and 24. These ranges are quite generous, and your target BMI should be toward the middle of them, say around 22. So put your finger on the BMI number 22 (shown in bold) and drop down until you reach your height, which is shown in the left margin. The number at that intersection is what your weight should be to achieve this BMI target.

Let's look at a couple of examples. Mary is 5 feet 6 inches and weighs 160 pounds. Her BMI is 26, which is 4 notches above her target BMI of 22. This means Mary has to lose 24 pounds in order to bring her to her 22 BMI goal of 136 pounds. Fred is 6 feet and weighs 190 pounds. His BMI is also 26, but he needs to lose 28 pounds to bring his BMI down to the 22 target of 162 pounds.

Another measurement that is important to know is your waist circumference. It indicates your level of abdominal fat, which is significant to your health, especially your heart health. People with a high level of abdominal fat, whom doctors describe as apple-shaped, have a much higher risk of developing cardiovascular disease and Type 2 diabetes (see chapter 9). To measure your waist, take a measuring tape and wrap it around your natural waist just above the navel. Don't be tempted to do a walk-down-the-beach-sucking-it-in routine. Just stand in a relaxed position and keep the measuring tape from cutting into your flesh. Your health is at risk if your waist circumference is 32 inches or more for women and 37 inches or more for men. A measurement of 35 inches plus for women and 40 inches plus for men puts you at high risk for a heart attack or stroke.

The 24 pounds that Mary has to shed and the 28 that Fred needs to lose are pounds of fat—Mary's and Fred's energy storage

BODY MASS INDEX (BMI)

	normal						overweight					obese		
BMI	19	20	21	**22**	23	24	25	26	27	28	29	30	31	32
height (inches)	body weight (pounds)													
58	91	96	100	**105**	110	115	119	124	129	134	138	143	148	153
59	94	99	104	**109**	114	119	124	128	133	138	143	148	153	158
60	97	102	107	**112**	118	123	128	133	138	143	148	153	158	163
61	100	106	111	**116**	122	127	132	137	143	148	153	158	164	169
62	104	109	115	**120**	126	131	136	142	147	153	158	164	169	175
63	107	113	118	**124**	130	135	141	146	152	158	163	169	175	180
64	110	116	122	**128**	134	140	145	151	157	163	169	174	180	186
65	114	120	126	**132**	138	144	150	156	162	168	174	180	186	192
66	118	124	130	**136**	142	148	155	161	167	173	179	186	192	198
67	121	127	134	**140**	146	153	159	166	172	178	185	191	198	204
68	125	131	138	**144**	151	158	164	171	177	184	190	197	203	210
69	128	135	142	**149**	155	162	169	176	182	189	196	203	209	216
70	132	139	146	**153**	160	167	174	181	188	195	202	209	216	222
71	136	143	150	**157**	165	172	179	186	193	200	208	215	222	229
72	140	147	154	**162**	169	177	184	191	199	206	213	221	228	235
73	144	151	159	**166**	174	182	189	197	204	212	219	227	235	242
74	148	155	163	**171**	179	186	194	202	210	218	225	233	241	249
75	152	160	168	**176**	184	192	200	208	216	224	232	240	248	256
76	156	164	172	**180**	189	197	205	213	221	230	238	246	254	263

Source: U.S. National Heart, Lung, and Blood Institute

							extreme obesity									
33	34	35	36	37	38	39	40	41	42	43	44	45	46	47	48	49
158	162	167	172	177	181	186	191	196	201	205	210	215	220	224	229	234
163	168	173	178	183	188	193	198	203	208	212	217	222	227	232	237	242
168	174	179	184	189	194	199	204	209	215	220	225	230	235	240	245	250
174	180	185	190	195	201	206	211	217	222	227	232	238	243	248	254	259
180	186	191	196	202	207	213	218	224	229	235	240	246	251	256	262	267
186	191	197	203	208	214	220	225	231	237	242	248	254	259	265	270	278
192	197	204	209	215	221	227	232	238	244	250	256	262	267	273	279	285
198	204	210	216	222	228	234	240	246	252	258	264	270	276	282	288	294
204	210	216	223	229	235	241	247	253	260	266	272	278	284	291	297	303
211	217	223	230	236	242	249	255	261	268	274	280	287	293	299	306	312
216	223	230	236	243	249	256	262	269	276	282	289	295	302	308	315	322
223	230	236	243	250	257	263	270	277	284	291	297	304	311	318	324	331
229	236	243	250	257	264	271	278	285	292	299	306	313	320	327	334	341
236	243	250	257	265	272	279	286	293	301	308	315	322	329	338	343	351
242	250	258	265	272	279	287	294	302	309	316	324	331	338	346	353	361
250	257	265	272	280	288	295	302	310	318	325	333	340	348	355	363	371
256	264	272	280	287	295	303	311	319	326	334	342	350	358	365	373	381
264	272	279	287	295	303	311	319	327	335	343	351	359	367	375	383	391
271	279	287	295	304	312	320	328	336	344	353	361	369	377	385	394	402

tanks. In order for them to lose weight, they must access and draw down those fat cells. This reminds me of a peculiar contraption used in England during World War II. The famous double-decker buses were converted to run on natural gas and had their upper deck changed into a natural gas tank, consisting of a large fabric balloon. When full, the balloon puffed up several feet above the top of the bus. As it proceeded along its route, the balloon slowly deflated, disappearing by the end of its destination, where it was reinflated. That's how I visualize our body fat: a deflating balloon from which we draw down our energy, except that in our case the balloon is around our waist, hips, and thighs!

So how do you draw down energy from your fat cells? By consuming fewer calories than your body needs. This will force your body to start using its fat stores to make up for the shortfall. Now, I know no one wants to hear about calories, particularly those of us who've tried long and hard to lose weight. Nevertheless, unless you are among those rare and blessed people whose metabolism and genetics enable them to eat as much as they want without gaining an ounce—and if you are, why would you be reading this book?—you, like me and the rest of us mere mortals, are doomed to the inevitable equation. But don't be disheartened. You can easily reduce your daily calorie intake without going hungry and without having to calculate the number of calories in everything you put in your mouth. All you have to do is eat low-G.I. foods (of course!) and adjust the ratio of carbohydrates, fats, and proteins in your diet.

Ultimately, all food is a source of energy for our bodies, and we measure energy in calories. The average adult uses somewhere between 1,500 and 3,000 calories a day, depending upon level of activity, rate of metabolism, and body weight. What people have been advised to do for decades is to get 55 percent of their calories from carbohydrates, 30 percent from fats, and 15 percent from protein. But with our more advanced knowledge of nutrition and how our digestive system works, this ratio is being challenged by many physicians and nutritionists. Accordingly, I recommend a modest adjustment to the traditional ratio. You should still get 55 percent of your calories from carbohydrates, but I am recommending that you eat less fat and a bit more protein than what has traditionally been advocated. A recent Harvard School of Public Health study involving more than eighty thousand women concluded that a moderately high level of protein intake (24 percent) is beneficial to heart health. Also, the more one exercises, the more protein one needs. Elite athletes require up to twice the amount of protein as the average person. Though I certainly don't expect you to become an elite athlete, I will be encouraging more exercise in chapter 8.

SOURCE OF CALORIES

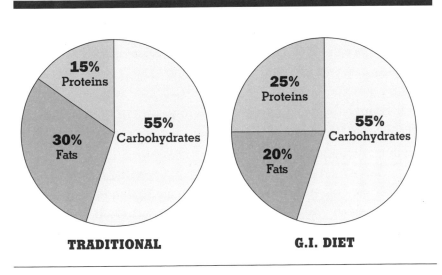

modest adjustment to the traditional ratio.

TRADITIONAL

G.I. DIET

Okay, so we now have the ratio that will help us to lose those extra pounds. It's all fine in theory, but what does it mean in the real world? That's what the rest of this book is all about: how much of what to eat, and when. I promised you a simple eating plan that reflects the real world we live in, and that is what I'll give you. The plan is divided into two phases. In Phase I, you'll be reducing your caloric intake, burning off those excess fat cells, and slimming down to a healthy, ideal weight. I recommend you target to lose **an average of 1 pound per week.** Some weeks, you will certainly lose more, especially in the early stages. Other weeks, you will probably plateau. So play the averages—1 pound per week. Phase I takes between three and six months, and for most people it's really a matter of simple math. A pound of fat contains around 3,600 calories. To lose that pound in one week, you must reduce your caloric intake by around 500 calories per day (500 x 7 days = 3,500 calories). So if you want to lose 20 pounds, it will take 20 weeks. Here's an example: Mark weighs 180 pounds and he wants to lose 18 pounds. In order to lose a pound a week, Mark must reduce his calorie consumption by 3,500 calories per week. Based on this, it will take Mark 18 weeks to lose 18 pounds. Take a look at the chart on the next page to get a sense of how long you should expect to be in Phase I of the G.I. Diet. Even if you don't find your exact weight and target weight, it will give you a good idea.

If twenty-five weeks seems like a long time to you, think of it in terms of the rest of your life. What's half a year compared with the many, many years you'll spend afterward with a slim, healthy body? This isn't a fad diet—fad diets don't work. The G.I. Diet is a wholesome and surefire route to permanent weight loss.

The reason I've included all this math is to help you understand this diet and how it's going to work for you. But I don't want you to think that you're going to have to do any calculations yourself! They're all built into the program. All you have to do is look at my food guide, which lists nearly every food that you can think of in one of three categories that are based on the colors of traffic lights. Foods listed in the red-light, or "stop," category are high-G.I. foods. They include bagels, watermelon, rice cakes, and melba toast, and they should be avoided. These foods are digested by your body so quickly that they are just not worth it. Foods in the yellow-light, or "caution," category—for example, muesli, corn, and bananas—raise your insulin levels to the point where weight loss is not going to happen, and should therefore also be avoided in Phase I. The foods that will make you lose weight are the ones that are listed in the green-light, or "go ahead," category. Fettuccine, basmati rice, grapes, and many, many others are all green-light foods. Eat them and watch your weight drop.

TARGET WEIGHT TIMETABLE

(Based on 10% Weight Reduction)

PRESENT WEIGHT	TARGET WEIGHT	WEEKS TO TARGET WEIGHT
120	108	12
130	117	13
140	126	14
150	135	15
160	144	16
170	153	17
180	162	18
190	171	19
200	180	20
210	189	21
220	198	22
230	207	23
240	216	24
250	225	25

When you've reached your target BMI, Phase II begins. Here, your caloric input and output are balanced. You're no longer trying to lose weight, so you can start eating foods from the yellow-light category from time to time. All you're doing at this point is maintaining your new weight.

So the two major obstacles to permanent weight loss, which I discussed at the beginning of the book—complicated instructions and feeling hungry or deprived—have both been addressed. The final part of the equation is you. The tools are at hand, but to make them work effectively takes motivation and a desire to succeed.

Are you ready? If so, let's get going with Phase I.

---

to sum up

1. Set a realistic weight-loss target. A BMI of 22 is the ideal goal.

2. In Phase I of the G.I. Diet, you'll be reducing the number of calories you consume by adjusting your caloric-intake ratio and by eating low-G.I., low-fat foods.

3. When you reach your target BMI, you'll start Phase II of the G.I. Diet, which evens out the number of calories you consume and expend.

Phase I

efore we go any further, I'd like you to do a little assignment. Try to remember as best you can what you've been eating over the past seven days and fill in the "current" columns of the chart on the next page. This exercise will give you a bit of a reality check and help you to form a baseline or starting point from which to build your new G.I. Diet program. Later in the book, I will ask you to return to this page and record what you've been eating for the past week. I think you'll find the change very interesting—even enlightening.

With the theory and science of the G.I. Diet behind us, it's time to get practical! As you know, Phase I is the weight-loss portion of the program, so we'll be sticking with low-G.I., low-fat foods, which are categorized as green. In most cases, you can eat as much of the green-light foods as you want. It's very important at this stage to eat frequently. This isn't a deprivation diet! So don't leave your digestive system with nothing to do. The saying "The devil finds work for idle hands" also applies to your stomach. If your digestive system is busy processing food and steadily supplying energy to your brain, you won't be looking for high-calorie snacks.

FOOD JOURNAL

DAY	BREAKFAST		LUNCH		DINNER		SNACKS	
	CURRENT	G.I. DIET	CURRENT	G.I. DIET	CURRENT	G.I. DIET	CURRENT	G.I. DIET
Monday								
Tuesday								
Wednesday								
Thursday								
Friday								
Saturday								
Sunday								

Don't skip breakfast. People who miss breakfast leave their stomachs empty from last night's dinner to lunch the next day—often more than sixteen hours! No wonder they gorge themselves at lunch and then look for a sugar fix mid-afternoon as they run out of steam. Always eat three meals a day—breakfast, lunch, and dinner—that contain approximately the same amount of energy (calories), as well as up to three snacks. *Never use sugar.* If you need a sweetener, use a sugar substitute such as Sweet'N Low or Equal. (There has been a considerable amount of negative publicity, generated principally by the sugar industry, about sweeteners. This has triggered dozens of studies worldwide, none of which has shown any long-term risks to our health. These products are safe and of real value in calorie control. But, as with most foods, don't go overboard. An excellent summary of the issue from the FDA can be found at www.fda.gov under "sugar substitutes.") And because liquids don't seem to trip our satiety mechanisms, don't waste your calorie allocation on beverages. Always drink water, skim milk, and other no-cal or low-cal beverages.

Portions

Understanding portions is essential if the G.I. Diet is to work for you. Since most vegetables and fruits have a low G.I. rating and are low in calories and fat, they are the most important food group in the G.I. Diet. However, both the U.S. and Canadian governments suggest that grains should be the most important food group. If you look at the U.S. Department of Agriculture's Food Pyramid on the next page, you will see that it suggests grains should be the largest component of your diet, followed by vegetables and fruit. But by giving grains priority, these governments and most nutritionists are promoting the leading cause of overweight and obesity. The Mayo Clinic has recently changed its Healthy Weight Pyramid to one where "fruit and vegetables are located at the bottom of the pyramid as opposed to the bread, cereal, and starch group because these foods are very low in calories and high

USDA FOOD PYRAMID

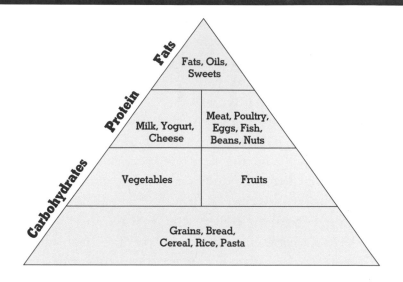

Source: U.S. Department of Agriculture

THE G.I. DIET FOOD PYRAMID

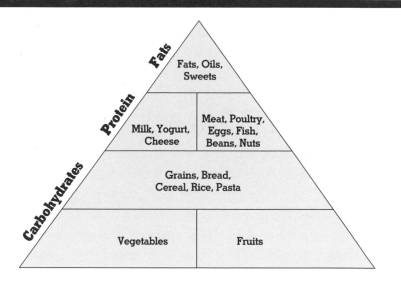

TRADITIONAL   G.I. DIET

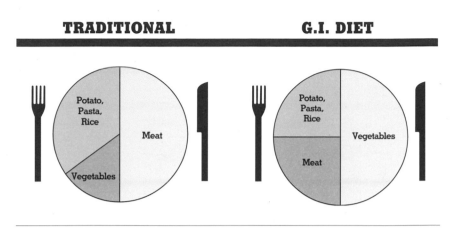

in health-enhancing properties." This is exactly what the G.I. Diet recommends, as you can see from the G.I. Diet Food Pyramid on the facing page.

To translate the pyramid to your dinner plate, dish out enough vegetables to cover 50 percent of your plate, enough meat, poultry, or fish to cover 25 percent of your plate, and enough rice, pasta, or potatoes to cover the remaining 25 percent. Don't bend the rules by piling your food too high!

At the top of this page are diagrams of the way we traditionally visualize our dinner plate and the healthier G.I. Diet version.

PHASE I MEALS

So now that you know about food portions, what can you eat? Let's talk about breakfast first. The following chart lists breakfast foods in the three color-coded categories. (For a comprehensive list, see Appendix I on page 125.) Following the chart is an explanation of how certain popular foods are categorized. If a food is not included in the chart, it is usually because a rating has not yet been established.

BREAKFAST

PROTEIN

	RED LIGHT	YELLOW LIGHT	GREEN LIGHT
meat/eggs	Regular bacon Regular eggs Sausages	Omega-3 eggs Turkey bacon	Canadian bacon/Lean ham Egg Beaters Egg whites Liquid eggs
dairy	Cheese Cottage cheese (whole or 2%) Cream Cream cheese Milk (whole or 2%) Sour cream Yogurt (whole or 2%)	Cheese (low-fat) Cream cheese (light) Milk (1%) Sour cream (light) Yogurt (low-fat with sugar)	Buttermilk Cheese (fat-free) Cottage cheese (1% or fat-free) Cream cheese (nonfat) Milk (skim) Sour cream (fat-free) Soy or whey protein powder Fruit yogurt (fat- and sugar-free)

CARBOHYDRATES

	● RED LIGHT	● YELLOW LIGHT	● GREEN LIGHT
cereals	All cold cereals except those listed as yellow or green light Cream of Wheat Granola Grits Instant/quick-cook oatmeal Muesli (commercial)	Post Shredded Wheat 'N Bran	All-Bran Bran Buds Fiber One Homemade Muesli (see page 72) Kashi Go Lean Large-flake oat-meal (e.g., Quaker Old-Fashioned Oats) Oat bran
breads/ grains	Bagels Baguettes Croissants Doughnuts English muffins Pancakes/Waffles Regular granola bars White bread	Whole-grain breads	Apple Bran Muffins (see page 93) Homemade Granola Bars (see page 95) 100% stone-ground whole wheat bread* Whole-grain, high-fiber bread*
fruits	All canned fruits in syrup All dried fruit Applesauce containing sugar Cantaloupe Melons Raisins	Apricots Bananas Fruit cocktail in juice Pineapple	Apples Applesauce (unsweetened) Grapefruit Grapes Oranges Peaches Pears Plums

*Use a single slice only per serving; 2½–3 grams of fiber per slice.

● RED LIGHT	● YELLOW LIGHT	● GREEN LIGHT
juices All fruit drinks All sweetened juices Prune Watermelon	Apple (unsweetened) Cranberry (unsweetened) Grapefruit (unsweetened) Orange (unsweetened) Pear (unsweetened) Pineapple (unsweetened)	Eat the fruit rather than drink its juice
vegetables* French fries Hash browns		Most vegetables*

*See page 125 for complete list.

FATS

● RED LIGHT	● YELLOW LIGHT	GREEN LIGHT
Butter Hard margarine Tropical oils Vegetable shortening	Soft margarine (nonhydrogenated) Vegetable oil	Almonds** Canola oil** Hazelnuts** Soft margarine (nonhyrdrogenated, light)**, e.g., Promise Ultra Olive oil**

**Limit portions (see page 56).

Juice/Fruit

• Always eat the fruit rather than drink its juice. Juice is a processed product that is more rapidly digested than the parent fruit. To illustrate the point, diabetics who run into an insulin crisis and are in a state of hypoglycemia (low blood sugar) are usually given orange juice, which is the fastest way to get glucose into the bloodstream. A glass of juice has two and a half times the calories of a fresh whole orange. The "flesh" of the fruit also contains fiber and other macronutrients such as minerals that aren't found in juice.

Cereals

• Large-flake or slow-cooking oats are the best choice for two reasons: Oatmeal stays with you all morning and it's great for your heart, as it lowers cholesterol. (The cooking time is only around three minutes in the microwave.) Oat bran is also excellent.

• Among cold cereals, go for the high-fiber products—the ones that have at least 10 grams of fiber per serving. Fiber content is clearly indicated on cereal packages.

• High-fiber cereals are a great base to which fruit, nuts, and yogurt may be added.

Dairy

• The beverage of choice is skim milk. I had a real problem with skim milk both on cereal and as a beverage, but I persevered. Move down from 2% to 1% to skim in stages. I find that 2% tastes like cream now!

• Yogurt is a real plus. But look for low-fat or nonfat versions and, just as important, look for the artificially sweetened products. (Aspartame is the most commonly used sweetener.) Regular low-fat yogurts have nearly twice the calories as the aspartame versions.

- Cottage cheese is an excellent and filling source of protein. Again, go for the 1% or fat-free variety. Add fruit or light fruit spreads for flavor.

- Use other dairy products sparingly. Avoid most cheeses as they are high in saturated fat, which heads straight for your arteries. The dairy industry has a lot to answer for when it comes to our health. The success of their massive cheese advertising and promotion campaigns, often aimed at children, is reprehensible. If cheese is your thing, then go for the nonfat options such as nonfat cream cheese, which is an excellent green-light product. Or use stronger-flavored ones, such as Stilton or feta, but only sprinkled sparingly as a flavor enhancer.

Bread

- Always choose 100% stone-ground whole wheat or whole-grain high-fiber-breads. Fiber is the important ingredient. Look for 2½–3 grams of fiber per slice. The standard serving for bread is often listed as two slices, but make sure you only have one slice. "Stone ground" is important because stones grind grain more coarsely than the steel rollers that grind most of our flour. The coarser the grind, the less the fiber is separated, resulting in a far lower G.I. rating.

Eggs

- Choose liquid eggs and egg whites which are virtually fat- and cholesterol-free. An excellent green-light food.

Spreads/Preserves

- Do not use butter. The latest premium brands of nonhydro-genated light soft margarine such as Promise Ultra are acceptable.

- In fruit spreads or preserves, look for the "double fruit, no added sugar" versions. These taste terrific and are remarkably low in calories. Avoid products that list sugar as the first ingredient.

Bacon

- Sorry, but regular bacon is a red-light food. Acceptable alternatives are Canadian bacon and lean ham.

Coffee/Tea

- Coffee ideally should be decaffeinated (see page 53). Never add sugar, and use only 1% or skim milk.

- Tea is acceptable, as it has considerably less caffeine than coffee.

LUNCH

Most of us eat lunch outside the home, so it can be the most problematic meal, limited by time, budget, and availability considerations. But there appears to be a trend to "brown-bag" lunch, which gives you considerably more control over your food options. I list some easy green-light recipes on page 77 under Meal Ideas. Here are some practical guidelines for when you bring lunch or eat out.

PROTEIN

	RED LIGHT	YELLOW LIGHT	GREEN LIGHT
meat/eggs	Bologna	Omega-3 eggs	Beef (lean cuts)
	Bratwurst	Ground beef	Chicken/turkey
	Ground beef	(lean—10–20%	breast (skinless)
	(regular—more	fat)	Egg Beaters
	than 20% fat)	Lamb (lean cuts)	Egg whites
	Regular eggs	Pork (lean cuts)	Ground beef
	Hamburgers		(extra lean—10%
	Hot dogs		or less fat)
	Pastrami		Lean deli ham
	Salami		Liquid eggs
	Sausages		Seafood, fresh or
			frozen (no batter
			or breading) or
			canned (in water)
			Smoked salmon
			Veal
dairy	Cheese	Cheese (low-fat)	Cottage cheese
	Cottage cheese	Cream cheese	(1% or fat-free)
	(whole or 2%)	(light)	Cream cheese
	Cream cheese	Milk (1%)	(nonfat)
	Milk (whole or	Yogurt (low-fat	Ice cream (low-
	2%)	with sugar)	fat and no added
	Yogurt (whole or		sugar)
	2%)		Milk (skim)
			Fruit yogurt (non-
			fat and sugar-free)

CARBOHYDRATES

	RED LIGHT	YELLOW LIGHT	GREEN LIGHT
breads/ grains	Baguettes/ Croissants Cake/Cookies Doughnuts Gnocchi Hamburger buns Macaroni and cheese Muffins Noodles (canned or instant) Pancakes/ Waffles Pasta filled with cheese and/or meat Pizza Rice (instant, short grain, white) Tortillas White bread	Pita (whole wheat) Tortillas (low-carb) Whole grain breads*	Pasta, preferably whole wheat (fettuccine, linguine, macaroni, penne, spaghetti, vermicelli) Rice (basmati, brown, long-grain, wild) 100% stone-ground whole wheat bread* Whole-grain, high-fiber bread*
fruits/ vegetables	All dried fruit French fries Melons Potatoes (mashed or baked) Raisins	Apricots Bananas Corn Kiwi Papaya Pineapple Potatoes (boiled)	Asparagus Beans (green/wax) Bell peppers Broccoli Cabbage Carrots Cauliflower Celery Cucumbers

*Use a single slice only per serving; 2½–3 grams of fiber per slice.

GREEN LIGHT

fruits/ vegetables (continued)		
Eggplant	Snow peas	Apples
Lettuce	Spinach	Applesauce
Mushrooms	Tomatoes	(unsweetened)
Olives*	Zucchini	Blackberries
Onions		Blueberries
Peas		Grapefruit
Pickles		Grapes
Potatoes (boiled, small, new)**		Oranges
		Peaches
		Pears
		Plums
		Raspberries
		Strawberries

FATS/CONDIMENTS

🔴 RED LIGHT	🟡 YELLOW LIGHT	GREEN LIGHT
Butter	Soft margarine (nonhydrogenated)	Almonds*
Hard margarine		Canola oil*
Ketchup	Mayonnaise (light)	Hummus
Mayonnaise	Most nuts	Mayonnaise (fat-free)
Salad dressings (regular)	Salad dressings (light)	Mustard
Tropical oils		Soft margarine (nonhydrogenated, light)*; e.g., Promise Ultra
Vegetable shortening		Olive oil*
		Salad dressings (fat-free)

*Limit quantity (see page 56).

**2 to 3 per serving.

SOUPS

RED LIGHT	YELLOW LIGHT	GREEN LIGHT
All cream-based soups Black bean Green pea Split pea Puréed vegetable	Chicken noodle Lentil Tomato	Chunky bean and vegetable soups (e.g., Campbell's Healthy Request and Healthy Choice)

Bread

- Sandwiches are probably the most popular choice for lunch in North America, and they usually have a high G.I. rating and are high in calories. But you don't have to cut sandwiches out of your diet. To lower their impact on your hips, choose sandwiches made with whole wheat or whole-grain bread, the coarser the better. Then take off the top layer of the bread and eat the sandwich open-faced. Watch out for mayonnaise—it's often a major component in egg, chicken, and tuna salads. Always ask for no mayo—unless it's nonfat. Also request no butter or margarine on bread. Hummus and mustard are good alternatives.

Fast Food

- The simple answer to "Should I visit fast-food outlets for lunch?" is NO! With few exceptions, fast food is loaded with saturated fat and calories, with rarely a gram of fiber in sight. For example, a Quarter Pounder with cheese hits you with just under 500 calories and more than half your day's quota of fat. Merely being in the presence of all those tempting burgers, fries, and shakes makes your challenges more difficult—so stay away if at all possible! I can assure you that after a few months on the G.I.

Diet even the idea of fast food will turn you off. With your face pressed to the window of any fast-food joint, you'll watch with amazement what the heavyweights are putting away—straight to their waists and hips. That could have been you!

If your alternatives are limited, here are some ways to successfully navigate through this gastronomic minefield:

Burgers: Dispose of the top of the bun and don't order cheese or bacon. Keep it as simple as possible.

Fries: DON'T. A medium order of McDonald's fries contains 17 grams of fat (mostly saturated), about 50 percent of your total daily allowance.

Milk shakes: DON'T. The saturated fat and calorie levels are unbelievable.

Salads: Go for them, as much as you like, but notice the flashing red light over most dressings. Always use light or low-fat dressings, as they have less than a third of the calories of regular dressings. Failing that, use oil and vinegar. Ask for your dressing on the side so you can control the quantity. Avoid Caesar salads, as their high-fat dressing can be disastrous.

Chicken: Chicken (skinless) is a popular and classic green-light food. However, never eat breaded and fried KFC-style chicken, as this loads up the fat and calories. Always eat open-faced chicken sandwiches or subs with lots of vegetables and no cheese or mayo. Make sure the chicken is grilled, not deep-fried.

Wraps: An increasingly popular alternative to the traditional sandwich is a wrap. Ask for whole wheat pita bread or low-carb tortillas. While regular tortillas are red light, low-carb tortillas, if available, are acceptable with high fiber and low fat. They're also great for brown-bagging. If you choose pita bread, have it split in half so it's a single layer.

Pizza: Pizza is red-light due to both its high-G.I. crust and the massive amount of saturated (bad) fat from the traditional cheese-based toppings. If you are fortunate enough to have a restaurant that will make you a custom pizza, then ask for a super-thin whole wheat crust, tomato sauce, lots of vegetables, fresh herbs, and some sliced chicken breast (and *no* cheese). You can also make this at home using a split whole wheat pita bread (half thickness) as the crust.

Submarines: Ask for a whole wheat roll, but, again, eat it open-faced. Avoid cheese and mayo unless they're low-fat. And also avoid Italian subs, with their layers of processed deli meats.

Fish/Shellfish: An excellent choice providing there's no batter or breaded coating.

Chinese: The two things to watch for are the rice and the sauces, especially the sweet ones, which are high in sugar. Rice is usually a problem, as most restaurants use a glutinous high-G.I. rice whose grains tend to stick together. So avoid it if you can.

Mexican: Along with unacceptably high levels of fat, especially saturated, most Mexican fast food also has extremely high sodium (salt) levels. Many meals contain enough salt for over half your total daily requirement! Excessive levels of salt boost blood pressure, which can in turn lead to heart attacks and stroke.

So, in the long run, it's best to avoid these fast-food outlets and save both your waistline and your health.

Pasta

- Though most pastas are found in the moderate G.I. category, they are a villain in our obesity problem, not because of any issue with pasta itself—a moderate-G.I. and low-fat (although high-calorie) product—but due to the quantities we eat. In Italy, they are aghast at the huge bowls of pasta we consume as our main course. They quite correctly view pasta as an appetizer or a side dish. We typically view it as the bulk of the meal, with sauce and a few pieces of protein on top.

  Because it's difficult when dining out to order a partial plate of pasta, it's best either to order a pasta entrée to split with a friend, or to ask for a to-go container to be delivered with the meal so that before you begin eating, you can put away the extra pasta for later and avoid the temptation of overeating. If you are able to obtain a side order, then limit the quantity to cover a quarter of the plate (about ¾ cup) and ask for low-fat sauce options. Please, no Alfredo. If whole-grain pasta is available, go for it.

Soups

- A chunky bean or vegetable soup followed by fish or chicken makes an ideal lunch. Beware of cream-based or puréed vegetable soups; they are high in fat and heavily processed, therefore red light all the way.

  Note: Commercial soups have a higher G.I. rating than those cooked at home from scratch, due to high-temperature processing.

Potatoes

- Potatoes are a mid- to high-level G.I. vegetable depending on their starch content and how they are prepared. Boiled whole small new potatoes have the lowest starch content and the lowest G.I. Conversely, baked potatoes have the highest. Since it's almost impossible to get plain, boiled new potatoes when eating out, always ask your waiter for double vegetables in lieu of potatoes. In four years, after hundreds of requests, I've never been refused.

Rice

- Eat basmati, brown, wild, or long-grain rice only, and in quantities to cover no more than a quarter of your plate. These rices contain a starch, amylose, that breaks down more slowly than other rices. Avoid rice if it's glutinous and sticky.

Eggs

- Always ask for an egg substitute or egg whites when dining out. The more vegetables you can incorporate into your egg dish, the better.

Dessert

- If you have time, a fat- and sugar-free fruit yogurt is terrific. Always eat some fruit. I keep a supply of apples, pears, peaches, and grapes, depending on the season, in my office. Stay away from most other desserts.

SNACKS

Because it's a bad idea to leave your stomach empty, snacks are an important part of the G.I. Diet. But I'm afraid you'll have to avoid the customary choices like muffins, cookies, and chips, all high-G.I. foods that are calorie-dense. Two hours after eating them, you've added a few more fat cells and are feeling hungry again. These foods are just not worth the trouble!

Phase I snacks include fruit, sugar-free nonfat yogurt, nonfat or 1% cottage cheese, and raw vegetables. You might also want to explore the world of nutrition bars. Stay away from the expensive high-carbohydrate, high-calorie sugar bars, choosing instead those that have a more balanced ratio of carbohydrates, fats, and proteins. Half a Balance bar is an excellent snack, and so are most bars that weigh between 50 and 65 grams and have around 200 calories. They should contain 20 to 30 grams of carbohydrates, 12 to 15 grams of protein, and only 5 grams of fat. *Check labels carefully.*

If you bake your own low-G.I. muffins and granola bars (the recipes are in chapter 6), they also make good snacks. You can freeze a batch or two and reheat them in the microwave.

Though many snacks and desserts are billed as fat- and sugar-free, they are in fact high-G.I. because often all they contain are highly processed grains: for example, fat- and sugar-free puddings and Jell-O and fat- and sugar-free muffins.

Try to incorporate a balance of carbohydrates, fats, and proteins into each snack. For example, have a few nuts or nonfat, sugar-free yogurt with a piece of fruit. Though achieving this balance with each snack can be difficult, especially when you're away from home, the effort is worth it.

● RED LIGHT	● YELLOW LIGHT	● GREEN LIGHT
Candy	Bananas	Almonds**
Cookies	Dark chocolate	Homemade
Crackers	(70% cocoa)	Apple Bran
Doughnuts	Ice cream (low-	Muffins (see
French fries	fat)	page 93)
Regular granola	Most nuts	Applesauce
bars	Popcorn (light,	(unsweetened)
Ice cream	microwave)	Canned peaches
Milk chocolate		or pears in juice
Muffins (commer-		or water
cial)		Cottage cheese
Popcorn (regular		(1% or fat-free)
microwave)		Food bars*
Potato chips		Hazelnuts**
Pretzels		Homemade
Raisins		Granola bars
Rice cakes		(see page 95)
Tortilla chips		Ice cream (low-
Trail mix		fat and no added
		sugar)
		Most fresh fruit
		Most fresh veg-
		etables
		Macadamia
		nuts**
		Fruit yogurt (fat-
		and sugar-free)

*Warning: Most so-called nutrition bars are high-G.I. and high-calorie, with a lot of quick-fix carbs. Look for 50- to 65-gram bars, around 200 calories, with 20 to 30 grams of carbohydrates, 12 to 15 grams of protein, and 5 grams of fat per bar. (Balance bars are good choices.)

**8 to 10 nuts per serving.

DINNER

Dinner, traditionally, is the main meal of the day—and the one where most of us blow our diet to shreds. Unlike breakfast and lunch, dinner doesn't usually have any time or availability constraints (although juggling our schedules along with our families' can sometimes make this a moot point).

The typical American dinner comprises three things: meat or fish; potato, pasta, or rice; and vegetables. Together, these foods provide carbohydrates, proteins, and fats, along with other minerals and vitamins essential to our health. Though a few people add a starter, many more add a dessert, which is a real minefield of waistline temptation!

Here's a note on cooking and its impact on the Glycemic Index value of foods: We cook food not only to improve taste and flavor, but also to make it more digestible. In essence, cooking is the first step in the digestion of foods, as it starts the process of breaking down food that your digestive system completes. Not surprisingly then, cooking generally increases the G.I. of foods, particularly high-starch foods such as pastas, potatoes, and rice. So you should slightly undercook foods. They should be "al dente," as the Italians say, with some firmness to the bite.

PROTEIN

	● RED LIGHT	● YELLOW LIGHT	● GREEN LIGHT
meat/eggs	Ground beef (regular)	Ground beef (lean)	Beef (lean cuts)
	Regular eggs	Omega-3 eggs	Ground beef (extra lean)
	Hamburgers	Lamb (lean cuts)	Chicken breast (skinless)
	Hot dogs	Pork (lean cuts)	Egg whites
	Processed meats		Lean deli ham
	Sausages		Liquid eggs
			Seafood, fresh or frozen (no batter or breading) or canned (in water)

	RED LIGHT	YELLOW LIGHT	GREEN LIGHT
meat/eggs (continued)			Sushi (see page 68) Tofu Turkey breast (skinless) Veal
dairy	Cheese Cottage cheese (whole or 2%) Milk (whole or 2%) Sour cream Yogurt (whole or 2%)	Cheese (low-fat) Yogurt (low-fat with sugar)	Cottage cheese (1% or fat-free) Ice cream* (low-fat and no added sugar) Milk (skim) Fruit yogurt (fat- and sugar-free)

CARBOHYDRATES

	RED LIGHT	YELLOW LIGHT	GREEN LIGHT
breads/ grains	Bagels Baguette/ Croissants Cake/Cookies Cornbread Couscous Gnocchi Macaroni and cheese Muffins/ Doughnuts Noodles (canned or instant) Pancakes/Waffles Pasta filled with cheese and/or meat	Pizza Rice (instant, white) Tortillas White bread Pita (whole wheat) Sourdough bread Tortillas (low-carb) Whole-grain breads	Beans (black, red, white) Pasta, preferably whole wheat (fettuccine, linguine, macaroni, penne, spaghetti, vermicelli) Rice (basmati, brown, long-grain, wild) 100% stone-ground whole wheat bread** Whole-grain, high-fiber bread**

*Limit quantity (see page 56).

**Use only a single slice per serving; 2½–3 grams of fiber per slice.

	RED LIGHT	YELLOW LIGHT	GREEN LIGHT
fruits / vegetables	French fries Melons Potatoes (mashed or baked)	Apricots Bananas Corn Kiwi Papaya Pineapple Potatoes (boiled) Asparagus Beans (green/wax) Bell peppers Broccoli Cabbage Carrots Cauliflower Celery Cucumbers Eggplant Lettuce Mushrooms Olives* Onions Peas Pickles Potatoes (boiled small new)** Snow peas Spinach Tomatoes Zucchini	Apples Applesauce (unsweetened) Blackberries Blueberries Cherries Grapefruit Grapes Oranges Peaches Pears Plums Raspberries Strawberries

*Limit quantity (see page 56).

**2 to 3 per serving.

FATS

● RED LIGHT	● YELLOW LIGHT	● GREEN LIGHT
Butter Lard Hard margarine Mayonaise Salad dressings (regular) Tropical oils Vegetable shortening	Soft margarine (nonhydrogenated) Mayonnaise (light) Most nuts Salad dressings (light)	Almonds* Canola oil* Hazelnuts* Olive oil* Soft tub margarine (nonhydrogenated, light; e.g., Promise Ultra)* Mayonnaise (fat-free) Salad dressings (fat-free)

SOUPS

● RED LIGHT	● YELLOW LIGHT	● GREEN LIGHT
All cream-based soups Black bean Green pea Pureed vegetable Split pea	Chicken noodle Lentil Tomato	Chunky bean, vegetable, and pasta soups (e.g., Campbell's Healthy Request, and Healthy Choice)

*Limit quantity (see page 56).

Meat/Fish

• Most red meat contains saturated (bad) fat, so it's important to buy lean cuts or trim off all the visible fat. A loin steak trimmed to only ¼ inch of fat can have up to twice the fat of a steak with no trim. Obviously, some cuts of meat have intrinsically higher fat content, and these should be avoided. The best beef cuts are top round, bottom round, eye of round, and round tip. Next best are top sirloin and tenderloin. Check with your butcher if in doubt.

- Chicken and turkey are excellent choices *provided all the skin is removed.*

- Seafood is also an excellent choice. Though certain fish, such as salmon, have a relatively high oil content, this oil is extremely beneficial to your health, especially your heart health.

- Broiling and grilling meat and fish are recommended methods, as they allow excess fat to drain off. Use a nonstick pan for stove-top cooking so that less fat is required. A vegetable oil spray is also a good idea, as you will use less fat as you cook.

- In terms of quantity, the best measure for meat or fish is your palm. The portion should fit into the palm of your hand and be about as thick. Another good visual is a pack of cards—so my friends with small palms tell me!

Note to Vegetarians: Most people I know who are vegetarian don't need to lose weight. My middle son is a vegetarian, and at 6 feet 5 inches and 160 pounds, he looks undernourished. But if you are a nonmeat eater and need to lose weight, the G.I. Diet is the program for you. All you have to do is continue to substitute vegetable protein for animal protein—something you've been doing all along. However, because most vegetable protein sources, such as beans, are encased in fiber, your digestive system may not be getting the maximum protein benefit. So try to add easily digestible protein boosters like tofu and soy protein powder.

Meat Substitutes

There are an increasing number of green-light alternatives to animal protein. Most of these are soy based, and soy is an excellent source of protein and is low in saturated fat. Even so, soy can be high in total fats, so make sure you look for lower-fat versions of soy-based products, especially soy beverages.

Tofu, which is made from compressed soy-milk curds, is also an ideal protein source. It can be purchased in various degrees of firmness depending on how you intend to use it: softer for soups and spread, firmer for marinating, grilling, or stir-frying. Firm tofu can have nearly three times as much protein and fat as soft tofu because it is more concentrated, so be careful how much you use.

Potatoes

- As mentioned earlier, potatoes have a G.I. range from moderate to high, depending on the type and how they are cooked and served. In the lowest G.I. category are boiled new potatoes, two to three per serving. (The G.I. for boiled new potatoes is 56, due to their low immature starch content, while baked have a G.I. of 84.) All other versions are strictly red light.

Pasta

- As mentioned earlier, the serving size is critical. Pasta should preferably be a side dish and not form the base of the meal. In other words, it should take up only a quarter of your plate. Whole wheat pasta, available at most natural food stores and increasingly in your local supermarket, is preferable. Allow 35–40 grams of dried pasta per serving or ¾ cup cooked.

- Ensure your meal contains 4 ounces of protein (seafood or meat) and at least 1 cup of vegetables.

Rice

- Rice has a broad G.I. range. The best choices are basmati, wild, brown, or long-grain. Again, serving size is critical. Allow 3 tablespoons of dry rice per serving or ⅔ cup cooked.

Vegetables/Salad

- This is where you can go wild! Eat as many vegetables and as much salad as you like. In fact, this should be the backbone of your meal. Virtually all vegetables are ideal. Try to have a side salad with your daily dinner.

- Watch out for salad dressings. Use only fat-free ones or a small amount of olive oil with vinegar or lemon juice.

- Serve two or three varieties of vegetables for dinner. Frozen bags of mixed, unseasoned vegetables are inexpensive and convenient.

- To preserve the full nutritional benefit, slightly undercook, and preferably steam, stir-fry, or microwave, vegetables.

Desserts

- This is one of the most troublesome issues in any weight-control program. Desserts usually look and taste great, but they tend to be loaded with sugar and fat—a real guilt-inducing situation! As the last course in most meals, desserts often fall into the "Should I or shouldn't I?" category.

The good news is that dessert should be a part of your meal. There are a broad range of green-light alternatives that taste great and are good for you. Virtually any fruit qualifies (though hold off on the bananas and pineapple for now), and there are numerous low-fat and sugar-free dairy products such as yogurt and ice cream. You won't be eating apple pie à la mode, but you could be enjoying unsweetened applesauce with yogurt, or even a meringue with fresh or frozen berries.

BEVERAGES

Water

The cheapest and best beverage choice is plain water. Since 70 percent of our body is made up of water, it's hardly surprising that drinking water is an important part of any dietary program. Most dietitians recommend eight glasses of water per day. This sounds a bit steep to me, and every time I make a conscious effort to comply, I find myself running for the bathroom every couple of hours!

If you set out to drink eight glasses, you end up consuming a great deal more than that. We take in a great deal of water when we consume other liquids such as soft drinks, milk in cereal, and the water that makes up the bulk of most fruits and vegetables. You easily take in several cups a day without even trying. As a rule of thumb, drink an 8-ounce glass of water *before* each meal and snack. Having your stomach partly filled with liquid before the meal means you will feel full more quickly, thus reducing the temptation to overeat.

Skim Milk

My personal preference of beverage is skim milk, at least with breakfast and lunch. It's an ideal green-light food, and since most lunches tend to be protein deficient, drinking skim milk is a good way of making up some of the shortfall.

Soft Drinks

If water is too boring for you, go for sugar-free soft drinks, preferably also caffeine-free (see below). Remember, the sugar in a drink is less satisfying than an equal quantity of sugar in food, so don't waste your caloric-intake quota.

Coffee

The principal problem with coffee is caffeine. Although caffeine doesn't represent a health hazard in itself, there is growing evidence that it interferes with insulin's effectiveness. As a result, the body produces more insulin, which reduces your blood sugar levels and makes you feel hungry. This is particularly the case for people who have a BMI of 30 or more. So in Phase I, NO CAFFEINE. That means drinking decaffeinated coffee—no hardship, given the delicious range of decaffeinated options available today.

As an experiment, I asked a group of dinner guests whether they preferred caffeinated or decaffeinated coffee. It split about fifty-fifty. I then served top-quality decaffeinated coffee to everyone and asked how they liked it. I received more applause from those who had asked for caffeinated than from the dedicated decaf aficionados! I rest my case.

Note: Judging from the number of e-mail messages I've received, coffee and caffeine are a major concern for many of you. If this is a deal breaker and you simply can't face the day without that morning cup to get you started, go for it (see *Living with the G.I. Diet*, page 101).

Tea

Tea has considerably less caffeine than coffee. Both black and green teas also contain an antioxidant property that appears to carry a significant heart health benefit. In fact, there are higher quantities of flavonoids (antioxidants) in tea than in any vegetable tested. Two cups of black or green tea have the same amount of antioxidants as seven cups of orange juice or twenty of apple juice. Maybe my ninety-three-year-old mother and her tea-drinking cronies are onto something.

So, tea in moderation is fine. If you are looking for alternative teas that are completely caffeine-free, there has been an explosion of flavored herbal and fruit options, though they don't have the antioxidant characteristics of real tea. In fact, as I'm writing this, I'm drinking English toffee tea—delicious! These teas are a lot of fun and taste great.

Iced tea is good, too, as long as no sugar is added. Pre-sweetened tea, whether bottled or homemade, is red-light.

Fruit Drinks/Juices

Fruit drinks contain a large amount of sugar, are calorie-dense, and definitely belong on the red-light list.

Fruit juices, which are 100 percent pure juice, are preferable, but as we discussed earlier, it is always better to eat the fruit than to drink its juice. Remember, the more work your body has to do to break down food, the better. There is nothing worse than an idle stomach!

Alcohol

I'm sure this is the section that most readers fast-forward to. Well, it's a good news, bad news story.

The good news is that alcohol in moderation (and we'll discuss moderation in chapter 7) is not only acceptable, but, as you'll learn later, can even be good for your health.

The bad news is that alcohol in general is a disaster for weight control. Alcohol is easily metabolized by the body, which means increased insulin production, a drop in blood sugar levels, and demand from the body for more alcohol or food to boost those sagging sugar levels. This is a vicious cycle that can play havoc with your weight-loss plans. To make things worse, most alcoholic drinks are loaded with empty calories.

So, NO ALCOHOL at all in Phase I.

SERVING SIZE

Some nutritionists contend that today's weight problems have as much to do with serving size as with the type of food we eat. There is a great deal of truth to this. The "Big Mac" mentality has permeated our thinking. If one serving tastes terrific, think how good two will taste! And who doesn't like to feel they're getting a great deal. Twice the fries for an extra quarter. Beat that!

A trip to the movies encapsulates the problem. All popcorn, drinks, and candy come in giant sizes only. The fast-food industry in particular has recognized our desire to treat ourselves when we eat out by ordering larger servings, and they do everything to encourage that tendency. Food is a relatively cheap commodity, especially when it is high in low-cost simple carbohydrates such as sugar and flour. That is why fast-food companies can offer bigger servings at little incremental cost either to themselves or to you.

There are two principal rules in the G.I. Diet with regard to serving size:

1. Eat as much of the green-light foods as you like, except where specific portions or servings are indicated. Specific portions are especially important in the case of foods that have a middle-range G.I. rating or are particularly calorie-dense.

2. Everything in moderation, so don't go overboard on quantities of anything. Some readers have asked if eating twelve apples a day or an entire tub of cottage cheese at one sitting is acceptable! It is not.

Here are recommended green-light servings:

GREEN-LIGHT SERVINGS

almonds, hazelnuts, and macadamia nuts	½ ounce (8 to 10 nuts)
avocado	¼ cup
bread	1 slice
ice cream (low-fat, no added sugar)	½ cup
margarine (light)	2 teaspoons
meat/fish/poultry	4 ounces (pack of cards)
oatmeal and other cereals	½ cup
oil	1 teaspoon
olives	4 to 5
pasta	¾ cup cooked (¼ of plate)
potatoes (small, new)	2 to 3
rice	⅔ cup cooked (¼ of plate)

As in most things, common sense should be your guide. This book promised to keep things simple and not to have you counting calories or using other complex ways to measure food. If anything was going to turn you off to a weight-loss program, it would be difficult formulas, weights, and measures. Accordingly, the serving sizes listed on the facing page are an average for people who have a BMI under 30. For those readers who have a BMI of 30 plus who find themselves really struggling, I would recommend increasing these serving sizes by up to 50 percent until your weight has moved below the 30 BMI mark. At that time, you should reduce serving sizes to the recommended average portions listed. Once you have achieved your target BMI, you will move to Phase II as outlined later in the book. It will just take you a little longer to achieve your goal.

To make the G.I. Diet work and to keep things simple, you have to do your part by using your own good judgment. As with juries and democracy, the common sense of the public should not be underestimated!

---

to sum up

1. In Phase I, eat exclusively green-light foods, i.e., those with a low glycemic and calorie rating.

2. Eat three principal meals of equal nutritional value per day plus up to three between-meal snacks.

3. Drink lots of water or other green-light fluids, including an eight-ounce glass before or with each meal and snack. And don't touch caffeine or alcohol until Phase II!

4. Moderation and common sense are your guides for determining serving portions.

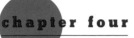

chapter four

Ready, Set, Go!

READY

I hope you understand the principles of the G.I. Diet by now and are totally convinced that the plan is worth a serious attempt, since it will be the way you (and your family) will eat for the rest of your life. All that's left is to take the plunge. This is what I call the ready stage, and it is perhaps the most difficult part of the journey.

(*Important note:* If you have any medical condition or are pregnant, check with your doctor before starting this or any diet plan.)

The best advice I can give comes from my own experience. I knew I had to lose 20 pounds to take me to the 22 BMI target weight. On the advice of a friend, I gathered together a number of books (diet books!) and piled them on my bathroom scale until they totaled 20 pounds. I then put them in a backpack and carried them around the house one Sunday morning. By noon, the weight was really bugging me. What a relief it was to take the bag off my back! So the question was, did I want to carry that excess 20 pounds of fat around with me each and every day, or lose it and gain the sense of lightness and freedom I experienced after the backpack came off?

I urge you to try the same exercise. Identify how much weight you want to lose by using the BMI chart on pages 18–19. Bundle up enough books to equal that weight and carry them on your back or shoulder or around your waist for a few hours. Remember, that's the excess weight you are permanently carrying around with you. No wonder you feel exhausted! That's one of the principal benefits of the G.I. Diet: Not only will you look and feel great, but you will find energy and zip you might have thought were long gone.

SET

Wondering what to do first? Well, let me suggest that you proceed in the following manner:

1. Baseline

Before you do anything else, get your vital statistics on record. Measuring progress is a great motivator. You will find a detachable log sheet on page 152 to keep in the bathroom so you can record your weekly progress. There are two key measurements. The first is weight. Always weigh yourself at the same time of day, because a meal or bowel movement can throw off your weight by a couple of pounds. First thing in the morning, before you eat breakfast, is a good time. The other important measurement is your waist. Measure at your natural waistline—usually just above the navel, while standing in a relaxed, normal posture. The tape should be snug but not indenting the skin.

Record both measurements on the bathroom log. I've added a "Comments" column to the log sheet, where you can note how you're feeling or any unusual events in the past week that might have some bearing on your progress.

2. Pantry

Clear out your pantry, fridge, and freezer of all red- and yellow-light products. Don't compromise; put them straight into the garbage—or better, donate them to an appropriate charitable organization. If these items are not around, you won't be tempted to eat or drink them.

3. Shopping

Stock up at home on products that get a green light. There is a Green-Light Kitchen Cupboard Essentials guide on page 133, and if you turn to page 135, you will find a detachable shopping list to take with you to the grocery store. After a couple of trips, selecting the right products will become second nature.

Although I've tried to provide a broad range of products, I could not hope to cover all the thousands of brands available in most supermarkets. This means you have to check labels when in doubt.

Reading Labels

For products and brands not specifically listed, look for the Nutrition Facts on the label. The key numbers to note are:

1. Serving size: Is this realistic? Often manufacturers who are concerned about the fat, cholesterol, or calories of that product will identify a serving size smaller than is realistic. Many high-sugar cereals do this.

2. Calories: A key number. Remember, it reflects the serving size, so again, check that the serving size is realistic.

3. Fat: Two numbers to note: total grams of fat and saturated fat. Again, these refer to the recommended serving size and therefore may be lowballing the real numbers. The number to be particularly concerned about is saturated, or "bad," fat. Unfortunately, hydrogenated oils, or trans fatty acids, are not indicated on food labels (and manufacturers have until the year 2006 to add that information).

4. Fiber: Dietary fiber is important, as most low-G.I. foods have a high fiber content. If it looks low, check if other brands are higher—4 to 5 grams per serving should be the minimum target.

There is a great deal more useful food information listed in the Nutrition Facts, but these four factors—serving size, calories, fat, and fiber—are the key ones to check, particularly when comparing one brand with another.

Basically, shop for foods that are low-sugar, low-fat (especially saturated), and high-fiber. That's the formula for all green-light products: They have a low G.I. and are calorie-light. By eating these foods, you will reduce your caloric intake without going hungry.

You will be buying considerably more fruit and vegetables than previously, so be a little daring and try some varieties that are new to you. There's a wonderful world of fresh and frozen produce just waiting for you to enjoy!

Caution: Don't go food shopping on an empty stomach, or you'll end up buying items that don't belong to the G.I. Diet!

GO

Now that you're on board with the G.I. Diet, the difficult part is done and it's plain sailing from here. Don't be surprised if you lose more than one pound per week in the first few weeks as your body adjusts to the new regimen. Some of that weight will be water, not fat. Remember, 70 percent of our body weight is water.

Don't worry if from time to time you "fall off the wagon," eating or drinking with friends and going outside the program. That's the real world, and though it will marginally delay your target date, it's more important that you not feel as though you're living in a straitjacket. I probably live about 90 percent within the program and 10 percent outside—by choice. I feel better and more energized when on the program and rarely feel deprived. However, in Phase I, try to keep these lapses to a minimum; you will be able to allow yourself more leeway once you have achieved your target weight. Keep reading for some motivating tips.

If you want further proof or reassurance that your new way of eating is really working, try this test. After eight weeks on the G.I. Diet, break all the rules and have a lunch consisting of a whole pizza with the works, a bread roll, and a beer or regular soft drink. While you're at it, finish up with a slice of pie. I'll spare you the ice cream.

I did just that, and by about three in the afternoon, I could hardly keep awake. I felt listless and worn out. I hadn't planned on eating so much but got caught up in a fellow employee's farewell lunch. The reason for my afternoon fatigue was the combination of high-G.I. foods (pizza, bread roll, beer, and pie), which led to a rapid spike in my blood sugar level. The resulting rush of insulin caused my sugar levels to drop precipitously, leaving my brain and muscles starved of energy—in a hypoglycemic state. No wonder I couldn't keep my eyes open.

Here are some tips to keep you motivated, especially when your resolve starts flagging (as it inevitably will from time to time):

1. Maintain a weekly progress log. (A removable log sheet appears on page 152.) Nothing is more motivating than success.

2. Set up a reward system. Buy yourself a small gift when you achieve a pre-determined weight goal—perhaps a gift for every three pounds lost.

3. Identify family members or friends who will be your cheerleaders. Make them active participants in your plan. Even better, find a friend who will join the plan for mutual support.

4. Avoid acquaintances and haunts that may encourage your old behaviors. You know who I mean!

5. Try adding what my friend calls a special "spa" day to your week—a day when you are *especially good* with your program. This gives you some extra credit in your weight-loss account to draw on when the inevitable relapse occurs.

To give you some encouragement and motivation as you start your journey, I'll leave you with the words of a few other readers who've found success with the G.I. Diet:

"I think this diet is amazing. I thought I would have problems giving up sugar, but I haven't at all. . . . I have lost just over ten pounds in a month, the most I have lost on any diet in years. To top it off, I feel great!" —Kathy

"I am thrilled about the fifty-pound weight loss (in just less than four months) and significant reduction in my blood sugar. After showing your book to many people, I think at least thirty copies have been purchased by my friends and family and even acquaintances." —Irene

"I know you hear this over and over again, but your book has done what I consider to be the impossible. Twenty weeks after going full-fledged into the program, I lost over thirty pounds and five inches off my waist! I'll continue your program for the rest of my life." —James

Sign up for the free G.I. Diet newsletter to learn from readers' experiences and keep up-to-date on the latest developments in diet and health. Details at **www.gidiet.com.**

---

to sum up

1. Try the weighted-backpack test (see page 58).
2. Take baseline weight and waist measurements.
3. Clear the pantry, fridge, and freezer of all red- and yellow-light products. Replace with green-light products.
4. Follow the five motivational tips (page 62) and do keep a record of your progress.
5. *Go for it!*

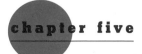
The Green-Light Glossary

The following is a summary of the most popular green-light foods. For a full green-light list, see Appendix I.

Apples A real staple. Use fresh for a snack or dessert. Unsweetened applesauce is ideal with cereals or with cottage cheese.

Barley An excellent supplement to soups.

Beans (legumes) If there's one food you can never get enough of, it's beans. These perfect green-light foods are high in protein and fiber and can supplement nearly every meal. Make bean salads or just add beans to any salad. Add to soups, replace some of the meat in casseroles, or add to meat loaf. Use as a side vegetable or as an alternative to potatoes, rice, or pasta. Check out the wide range of canned and frozen beans.

Exercise caution with baked beans, as the sauce can be high-fat and high-calorie. Check label for low-fat versions and watch your serving size.

Beans have a well-deserved reputation for creating "wind," so be patient until your body adapts—as it will—to your increased consumption.

Bread Most breads are red light except for coarse or stone-ground, 100% whole wheat or whole-grain breads. Check labels carefully, as the bread industry likes to confuse the unwary. "Stone-ground 100% whole wheat" is the wording to look for. With other breads, look for at least 2½ to 3 grams of fiber per slice.

Most bread is made from flour ground by steel rollers that strip away the bran coating. Stone-ground flour retains more of its bran coating, so it is digested more slowly in your stomach.

Even with stone-ground, 100% whole wheat bread, watch your quantity—one slice per serving. Use sparingly where you cannot avoid it, such as lunch in Phase I, and only occasionally in Phase II.

Cereals Use only large-flake oats, oat bran, or high-fiber cold cereals (10 grams of fiber per serving or higher). Though these cereals are not much fun in themselves, you can dress them up with fruit (fresh, frozen, or canned) or with fruit-flavored fat- and sugar-free yogurt. This way, you can change the menu daily. Use sweetener, not sugar.

Cottage cheese Fat-free or 1% cottage cheese is an excellent low-fat, high-protein food. Add fruit to make a snack or add it to salads.

Eggs By far the best options are egg whites or eggs in liquid form (packaged in a carton), which are virtually cholesterol- and fat-free. In Phase II, if you'd really rather use whole eggs, buy the omega-3 kind. The omega-3 content is beneficial for heart health.

Food Bars Most food or nutrition bars are a dietary disaster, high in carbohydrates and calories but low in protein. These bars are quick sugar fixes on the run. There are a few, such as Balance, that have a more equitable distribution of carbohydrates, proteins, and fats. Look for 20 to 30 grams of carbohydrates, 10 to 15 grams of protein, and 4 to 6 grams of fat. This equals about 220 calories per bar.

Serving size for a snack is one half of a bar. Keep one in your office desk or your purse for a convenient on-the-run snack. In an emergency, I have been known to have one bar plus an apple and a glass of skim milk for lunch when a proper lunch break was impossible. This is okay in emergencies, but don't make a habit of it.

Grapefruit One of the top-rated green-light foods. Eat as often as you like.

Hamburgers These are acceptable but only with extra-lean ground beef that has 10 percent or less fat. Mix in some oat bran to reduce the meat content but keep the bulk. A better option would be to replace the beef with ground turkey or chicken breast. Keep the serving size at 4 ounces; use only half of a whole wheat bun and eat open-faced.

Ice Cream Look for low-fat, no-sugar-added varieties, with 90 to 100 calories per ½-cup serving. And stick to this maximum serving size despite the temptation!

Milk Use skim only. If you have trouble adjusting, then use 1% and slowly wean yourself off it. The fat you're giving up is saturated (bad) fat. Milk is a terrific snack or meal supplement. I drink two glasses of skim milk a day, at breakfast and lunch.

Nuts A principal source of "good" fat, which is essential for your health. Almonds are your best choice. Add them to cereals, salads, and desserts. As they are calorie-dense, use in moderation.

Oat Bran An excellent high-fiber additive to baking as a partial replacement for flour. Also great as a hot cereal.

Oatmeal If you haven't had oatmeal since you were a kid, now's the time to revisit it. Large-flake or old-fashioned oatmeal is the breakfast of choice, with the added advantage for your heart of lowering cholesterol. A somewhat cynical colleague recently decided to take my advice about the G.I. Diet, but only a meal at a time, starting with oatmeal for breakfast. His oatmeal-based green-light breakfast has so far netted him ten pounds of weight loss! He's since thrown caution to the wind and is now a convert to three green-light meals a day. Personally, I often have hot oatmeal with unsweetened applesauce and sweetener as a snack on weekends.

Oranges Whole or in segments, fresh oranges are excellent as snacks, on cereal, and especially at breakfast. A glass of orange juice has two and a half times as many calories as a whole orange, so avoid the juice and stick with the real thing.

Pasta There are two golden rules. First, do not overcook; *al dente* (some firmness to the bite) is important. Second, serving size is key; pasta is a side dish and should never occupy more than a quarter of your plate. It *must not* form the basis of the meal, as it most commonly does nowadays in America, with disastrous results for waist-lines and hips. Whole wheat pasta is preferable.

Peaches/Pears Terrific snacks, desserts, or additions to break-fast cereal. Fresh, or canned in juice or water (not syrup).

Potatoes The only form of potatoes that is acceptable even on an occasional basis is boiled new potatoes. New potatoes have a low starch content, unlike larger, more mature potatoes that have been allowed to build their starch levels. All other forms of potato—baked, mashed, or fried—are strictly red light. Limit the quantity to two or three per serving.

Rice There is a wide range in the G.I. ratings for various types of rice, most of which are red light. The best rice is basmati or long grain, which is readily available at your supermarket. Brown rice is better than white. If rice is sticky, with the grains clumping together, don't use it. Similarly, don't overcook rice; the more it's cooked, the more glutinous and therefore unacceptable it becomes. The rule, then, is eat only slightly undercooked basmati rice.

Root Vegetables Most root vegetables, such as yams, sweet potatoes, beets, parsnips, and rutabaga, are red or yellow light, principally because of their high starch content. Accordingly, yellow-light root vegetables should be used in moderation in Phase II. However, carrots, with their low carbohydrate content, are green light.

Soups I recommend that all soups be made from scratch, as commercial soups are subjected to high temperatures in the canning process to kill bacteria, which raises the G.I. If convenience is important, then the brands listed in Appendix III are the best choices among the commercial soups.

Sushi Fish is an excellent green-light food. However, the rice normally served with sushi is glutinous and high-G.I. So eat the fish, but minimize the rice—stick with the sashimi options on the menu. If preparing at home, use basmati or long-grain rice. Prepared sushi rolls with their high rice content are not a good idea.

Sweeteners There has been a tremendous amount of misinformation circulating about artificial sweeteners—all of which has proven groundless. The sugar industry rightly sees these products as a threat and has done its best to bad-mouth them. Use sweeteners such as Splenda, Equal, Sweet'N Low, and Sugar Twin to replace sugar wherever possible. If you are allergic to sweeteners, then fructose is a better alternative than sugar.

Tofu Though not flavorful in itself, tofu is an excellent low-fat source of protein. Use it to boost or replace meat or seafood in dishes such as salads, burgers, and stir-fries.

Yogurt Fat- and sugar-free fruit-flavored yogurt is a near-perfect green-light product. It's an ideal snack food on its own, or a flavorful addition to breakfast cereal—especially hot oatmeal—and to fruit for dessert. Our fridge is always full of it, in half a dozen delicious flavors. In fact, my shopping cart is usually so full of yogurt containers that fellow shoppers frequently stop me to ask if they are on special!

Yogurt Cheese A wonderful substitute for cream in desserts or in main dishes like chili (see box on page 91).

Note: Additional green-light food updates can be found at **www.gidiet.com.**

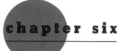

chapter six

Meal Ideas

When I wrote the first draft of this book, I neglected to include any recipes. My wife read the manuscript and suggested that readers would find them useful, especially when getting started on the diet. Since following the G.I. Diet requires you to change how you normally eat, she felt that including recipes would give you examples so you could adapt your own favorites to make them green light. She suggested that my lack of enthusiasm for including any had more to do with my own culinary incompetence than with any pedagogical stratagems (quite true).

So, stung into action and under her direction, I decided to offer recipes for the three primary meals and snacks for Phase I of the G.I. Diet. I have tried to adapt meal choices that are commonly eaten by most of us, so there is no need to worry about the unfamiliar. In these recipes, I have not only used green-light foods but also kept the use of fats in cooking down to a minimum. Always cook in nonstick pans, since they allow you to use only a small amount of fat when preparing food. Use a teaspoon or two of either canola or olive oil, or even better, use a vegetable oil cooking spray. Remember, there are 2,000 calories in 1 cup of oil, and fat in meat is high in cholesterol. Thus, grilling and broiling are excellent ways of cooking meat, since the fat from the meat drops into the pan or onto the coals.

Cutting fat doesn't mean you have to cut flavor or lose that all-important taste sensation. Cream products can be replaced by nonfat yogurt, yogurt cheese (see box on page 91), or fat-free sour cream. Use fat-free mayonnaise in tuna or chicken salads. You can still eat cheese, especially the strongly flavored ones like aged Cheddar, feta, blue cheese, and Gorgonzola, *but crumble and sprinkle it sparingly as a flavor enhancer only*, rather than using it as the prime ingredient. Try some new spices and flavored vinegars. Tomato salsa will spice up many foods without adding calories or fat, and fresh ginger adds life to stir-fries.

BREAKFAST

The first meal of the day is an important one, and oatmeal is the king of breakfast food. It is low-G.I. and low-calorie, is easy to prepare in the microwave, and stays with you all morning. Always use old-fashioned large-flake rolled oats—not one-minute or instant oats, as they have already been considerably processed. The body has to work harder to metabolize rolled oats, and this slows the digestive process and leaves you feeling fuller longer.

Oatmeal can be endlessly varied by changing the flavor of the fruit yogurt you add or by mixing in sliced fruit or berries. My wife's favorite way to eat oatmeal is with skim milk, unsweetened applesauce, sliced almonds, and sweetener.

Here's a recipe for my favorite oatmeal. Top it off with an orange and a glass of skim milk and you have a delicious breakfast that will stay with you all morning.

I've also included quick and easy suggestions for making your own muesli and improving cold cereal—fiber's never been so much fun! And you'll find a recipe for a basic omelet and four delicious green-light variations.

Oatmeal

1 serving

> *½ cup old-fashioned rolled oats*
> *1 cup water or skim milk*
> *½ to ¾ cup fat-free fruit yogurt with sweetener*
> *2 tablespoons sliced plain almonds*
> *Fresh fruit*

Place the oats in a microwave-safe bowl and cover with water or skim milk. Microwave the oats on medium power for 3 minutes. Mix in the yogurt, almonds, and some fresh fruit.

Homemade Muesli

2 servings

> *1 cup old-fashioned rolled oats*
> *¾ cup skim milk*
> *¾ cup fat-free fruit yogurt with sweetener*
> *2 tablespoons sliced plain almonds*
> *¾ cup berries or diced apple or pear*
> *Sweetener*

Place the oats in a bowl, cover them with the milk, and let soak in the refrigerator overnight. Add the yogurt, almonds, fruit, and sweetener to taste, and mix well.

Cold Cereal

1 serving

> *¾ cup wheat bran, such as All-Bran or Bran Buds*
> *¾ cup skim milk*
> *2 tablespoons sliced plain almonds*
> *¾ cup sliced peach or pear, or berries*
> *Sweetener*

Place the wheat bran in a bowl and pour the milk over it. Top with the almonds and fruit and add sweetener to taste.

Variation: A tasty alternative is to add ½ cup fruit-flavored fat-and sugar-free yogurt and to cut back a little on the milk. Though bran-based cereals are not a lot of fun in themselves, they are tasty when you add some fruit, nuts, and yogurt.

---

cooking with sweetener

Sweet'N Low, Equal (or their generic equivalents), and Splenda can all be substituted for sugar. These sweeteners are available in several forms—individual packets, baking granules, liquid, and tablets. While packets are generally equivalent in sweetness to 2 teaspoons of sugar, the intensity of sweetness can vary depending on the brand and the form, so check the label. If you are sweetening a beverage or ready-to-eat meal, simply use your own taste as a guide. If you are substituting for sugar in baking, follow the instructions on the box or the product Web site.

On-the-Run Breakfast

1 serving

> *1 cup sliced fresh fruit, such as apple, pear, peach,*
>   *strawberries, or blueberries*
> *½ cup cottage cheese (1% or fat-free)*
> *½ cup wheat bran, such as All-Bran or Bran Buds*
> *2 tablespoons sliced plain almonds*
> *1 slice toast, spread with 2 teaspoons margarine (light) and*
>   *1 tablespoon double-fruit, low-sugar preserves*

Place the fruit in a bowl and top with the cottage cheese, wheat bran, and almonds. Serve the toast alongside, and enjoy with a cup of decaffeinated coffee or tea.

Basic Omelet and Variations

1 serving

Omelets are easy to make, and you can vary them by adding any number of fresh vegetables, a little cheese, and/or some meat. You'll find the ingredients for a basic omelet here, along with suggestions for making Italian, Mexican, vegetarian, and Western versions. Don't stop with these—using the proportions as a guide, you can add whatever green-light ingredients strike your fancy. To round out the meal, include a cup of fresh fruit and a cup of skim milk or ½ to ¾ cup of fat- and sugar-free yogurt.

> *Vegetable oil cooking spray (preferably canola or olive oil)*
> *½ cup liquid eggs*
> *¼ cup skim milk*

Italian Omelet

½ cup sliced mushrooms
1 ounce grated skim mozzarella cheese
½ cup tomato puree
Chopped fresh or dried herbs, such as oregano or basil

Mexican Omelet

1 cup chopped red and green bell pepper
½ cup sliced mushrooms
½ cup canned beans, drained and rinsed
Hot sauce or chili powder, for sprinkling over the omelet (optional)

Vegetarian Omelet

1 cup small broccoli florets
½ cup sliced mushrooms
½ cup chopped red and green bell pepper
1 ounce grated skim-milk cheese

Western Omelet

1 cup chopped red and green bell pepper
1 small onion, chopped
2 slices Canadian bacon, lean deli ham, or turkey breast, chopped
Red pepper flakes or cayenne pepper (optional), for sprinkling over
the omelet

Omelet Preparation

1. Spray oil in a small nonstick skillet, then place it over medium heat.

2. Add the mushrooms, bell pepper, broccoli, and/or onion (depending on which omelet you are making), and sauté until tender, about 5 minutes. Transfer the sautéed vegetables to a plate and cover with aluminum foil to keep warm.

3. Beat the eggs with the milk and pour them into the skillet over medium heat. Cook until the eggs start to firm up, then spread the appropriate vegetables, cheese, herbs, beans, and/or meat over them. Continue cooking until the eggs are done to your liking.

4. If desired, sprinkle the omelet with hot sauce, chili powder, red pepper flakes, or cayenne, then serve.

Variation: Make scrambled eggs by stirring the eggs as they cook, adding any additional ingredients while the eggs are still soft.

LUNCH

If you are eating lunch out, refer to pages 39–43 for helpful tips about restaurants, take-out, and fast-food options. However, brown-bagging—bringing lunch to work—is becoming an increasingly popular option. This allows you to control what's in your lunch, plus you save money. If you already make your own lunch in advance at home, more often than not you'll find these lunches are short on protein and fiber.

Here are a few modifications and upgrades that will turn your brown-bag into a green-bag lunch. They will ensure that you feel full and energized for the afternoon. Just add fresh or canned fruit (in water, not syrup), plus a glass of water or (preferably) skim milk, and you've got yourself a lunch!

Basic Salad

1 serving

1½ cups torn or coarsely chopped lettuce and/or greens, such as romaine, leaf, Boston, or iceberg lettuce, mesclun, arugula, or watercress
1 small carrot, grated
½ red, yellow, or green bell pepper, chopped
1 plum tomato, cut into wedges
½ cup sliced cucumber
¼ cup sliced red onion (optional)
Basic Vinaigrette (recipe follows)

Place the lettuce and/or greens, carrot, bell pepper, tomato, cucumber, and onion, if using, in a bowl and toss to mix. Pour about 1 tablespoon of the vinaigrette over the salad and toss to mix.

Variations: Salads are green-light with plenty of fiber, but they don't usually have a lot of protein. Adding 4 ounces of canned tuna, cooked salmon, tofu, beans, chickpeas, cooked chicken, or another lean meat will provide a delicious solution to the problem.

Pay attention to the salad dressing. If you want to use a store-bought dressing, look for low-fat or fat-free.

Basic Vinaigrette

4 servings

> *2 tablespoons vinegar, such as white or red wine, balsamic,*
>   *rice, or cider, or lemon juice*
> *1 tablespoon extra-virgin olive oil or canola oil*
> *½ teaspoon Dijon mustard*
> *Pinch of salt*
> *Pinch of black pepper*
> *Pinch of dried herbs, such as thyme, oregano, basil,*
>   *marjoram, or mint, or Italian seasoning*

Place the vinegar, oil, mustard, salt, pepper, and herbs in a small bowl and whisk to combine.

Variation: Minced fresh herbs, such as Italian (flat) parsley or basil, make great additions to salads and vinaigrettes.

Storage: Both the salad and the vinaigrette can be prepared ahead and stored separately, covered, in the refrigerator for up to 2 days.

Salade Niçoise

1 serving

2 small new potatoes, cooked and quartered
1 cup green beans, briefly cooked
1 cup torn or coarsely chopped lettuce
1 tablespoon store-bought fat-free mustard vinaigrette
2 ounces canned tuna, drained and flaked
1 omega-3 egg, hard-boiled, peeled, and quartered
6 pitted black olives
1 medium tomato, quartered
1 anchovy fillet (optional)
Chopped fresh parsley
Salt and black pepper

Place the potatoes, beans, and lettuce in a bowl. Add the fat-free mustard vinaigrette and toss gently. Top with the tuna, egg, olives, tomato, and anchovy, if using. Sprinkle parsley on top, then season with salt and pepper to taste.

Variation: Substitute grilled fresh fish for the canned tuna.

Waldorf Chicken and Rice Salad

1 serving

¾ cup cooked basmati or brown rice
1 medium apple, chopped
1 or 2 stalks celery, chopped
¼ cup walnuts
4 ounces cooked chicken (page 83), chopped
1 tablespoon store-bought light buttermilk dressing

Place the rice, apple, celery, walnuts, and chicken in a bowl. Pour the buttermilk dressing on top and stir to mix. Keep refrigerated until lunch and enjoy.

Basic Pasta Salad Lunch

1 serving

½ to ¾ cup cooked whole wheat pasta (spirals,
*　shells, or similar shape)*
1 cup chopped cooked vegetables (such as broccoli,
*　asparagus, bell peppers, or scallions)*
¼ cup light tomato sauce or other low-fat
*　or nonfat pasta sauce*
4 ounces chopped cooked chicken (page 83)
*　or other lean meat, such as ground lean turkey*
*　or lean chicken sausage*

Place the pasta, vegetables, tomato sauce, and chicken in a bowl and stir to mix well. Refrigerate the salad, covered, until ready to use, then heat it in the microwave or serve chilled.

Variation: You can use the proportions here as a guide and vary the vegetables, sauce, and source of protein to suit your tastes and add variety to your pasta salad lunches.

sandwiches

The variations are endless, but here are some guidelines to make even the humble sandwich a convenient and filling green-light meal.

1. Always use stone-ground whole wheat or whole-grain high-fiber bread.

2. During Phase 1, sandwiches should be served open faced.

3. Include at least three vegetables, such as lettuce, tomato, red or green bell pepper, cucumber, sprouts, or onion.

4. Use mustard or hummus as a spread on the bread. No regular mayonnaise or butter.

5. Add 4 ounces of cooked lean meat or fish.

6. Mix tuna or chopped cooked chicken with low-fat mayonnaise or salad dressing and celery.

7. Mix canned salmon with malt vinegar (don't worry about bones)—a popular sandwich choice in Canada and the United Kingdom.

8. To help sandwiches stay fresh, not soggy, pack the components separately and assemble them just before eating, if possible.

Cottage Cheese and Fruit

1 serving

Perfect for a lunch on the run.

1 cup low-fat cottage cheese
1 cup chopped fresh fruit or fruit canned in juice,
such as peaches, apricots, or pears

Place the cottage cheese and fruit in a plastic bowl with a fitted lid, and stir to mix. Store in the refrigerator until lunchtime. Enjoy.

Variation: Add a tablespoon of double fruit, no added sugar fruit spread, or preserves instead of the chopped fruit.

DINNER

All of the following ideas for meals are based on the G.I. Diet portion ratios discussed in chapter 3. Vegetables should take up 50 percent of your plate and should ideally comprise at least one green vegetable, a mixture of at least two other vegetables, and a green salad. Meat, poultry, or fish should fill 25 percent of your plate, and rice, pasta, or potatoes should cover the remaining 25 percent.

I have based these meal ideas on typical family needs, modifying them according to G.I. principles.

Poultry: Basic Preparation

1 serving

Naturally low in fat, cooked chicken or turkey breast can be used in dozens of ways, combined with a variety of herbs, spices, and vegetables to enhance its flavor. You'll find instructions for a basic green-light method of cooking poultry here, followed by three recipes that use the cooked meat. The proportions are for one serving and can be multiplied as necessary for the recipes that follow.

> *Vegetable oil cooking spray (preferably canola or olive oil)*
> *4 ounces skinless, boneless chicken breast or turkey breast, whole, sliced, or cubed*

1. Spray oil in a small nonstick skillet, then place it over medium-high heat.

2. Add the chicken or turkey breast and sauté until firm to the touch and no longer pink, about 4 minutes per side for 1 chicken breast or piece of turkey or 5 to 6 minutes for slices or cubes.

Asian Stir-Fry

2 servings

> *Vegetable oil cooking spray (preferably canola or olive oil)*
> *3 cups chopped mixed vegetables, such as carrots, cauliflower,*
> *broccoli, mushrooms, and snow peas (see Note)*
> *1 teaspoon grated fresh ginger*
> *1 teaspoon soy sauce*
> *Salt and black pepper*
> *8 ounces cooked skinless, boneless chicken breast or turkey breast*
> *(page 83)*

1. Spray oil in a nonstick skillet, then place it over medium heat.

2. Add the mixed vegetables and sauté until tender, about 5 minutes.

3. Add the ginger and soy sauce and stir to mix. Season to taste with salt and pepper.

4. Add the cooked chicken or turkey and stir to mix. Let simmer until the chicken or turkey is heated through, 2 minutes, then serve.

Variation: To put the stir-fry together even more quickly, use 2 to 3 teaspoons of a light, store-bought stir-fry sauce in place of the fresh ginger, soy sauce, and salt and pepper.

Note: For color, add chopped mixed green, yellow, and red bell pepper. For convenience, use frozen mixed vegetables or frozen cut peppers.

Italian Chicken

2 servings

8 ounces sliced mushrooms
1 medium onion, sliced
1 can (18 ounces) chopped Italian tomatoes
1 clove garlic, minced
Chopped fresh or dried oregano and basil
8 ounces cooked skinless, boneless chicken breast or turkey breast
    (page 83)

1. Place the mushrooms, onion, and tomatoes in a saucepan. Stir in a little water, to prevent the tomatoes from sticking, and heat over medium-low heat until the mushrooms and onion are softened.

2. Add the garlic, oregano, and basil, stir to mix, then let simmer for 5 minutes.

3. Add the cooked chicken or turkey and stir to mix. Let simmer until the chicken or turkey is heated through, 2 minutes, then serve.

Chicken Curry

2 servings

Vegetable oil cooking spray (preferably canola or olive oil)
1 medium onion, sliced
1 to 2 tablespoons curry powder, or more to taste
1 cup sliced carrots
1 cup chopped celery
½ cup uncooked basmati rice
1 medium apple, chopped
¼ cup raisins
4 ounces cooked skinless, boneless chicken breast or turkey breast
  (page 83)

1. Spray oil in a nonstick skillet, then place it over medium heat.

2. Add the onion and curry powder, stir to coat the onion with the curry, then sauté for 1 minute.

3. Add the carrots and celery, stir to mix, then sauté for 1 minute.

4. Add the rice, apple, raisins, and 1 cup of water and stir to mix. Cover the skillet and let the curry simmer until all of the liquid is absorbed.

5. Add the cooked chicken or turkey and stir to mix. Keep over heat until the chicken or turkey is heated through, 2 minutes, then serve.

Fish: Basic Preparation

1 serving

Virtually any fish is suitable, but *never* use fish that is commercially breaded or in a batter. Salmon and trout are both great favorites at my house. Pre-spiced or flavored fish are okay, but why pay someone else a whopping premium for what you can easily do yourself? Here are directions for cooking a fish fillet in a microwave oven. It couldn't be easier. Proportions are for one serving and can be multiplied as necessary.

1 fish fillet (4 to 5 ounces)
1 to 2 teaspoons fresh lemon juice
Black pepper

1. Place the fish fillet in a microwave-safe dish.

2. Sprinkle the lemon juice and a dash of pepper over the fish.

3. Cover the dish with microwave-safe plastic wrap, folding back one corner slightly to allow the steam to escape.

4. Microwave the fish on high power until it is opaque in color and flakes when a fork is inserted, 4 to 5 minutes, rotating the dish 45 degrees halfway through cooking. Let stand for 2 minutes, then serve.

Variations

Sprinkle the fish with fresh or dried herbs, such as dill, parsley, basil, and/or tarragon.

Cook the fish on a bed of sliced leeks and onions. (Do not add oil).

Sprinkle the fish with a mixture of whole wheat bread crumbs and chopped parsley (1 tablespoon per fillet) combined with 1 teaspoon melted light nonhydrogenated margarine.

a green light for side dishes

Need some ideas for what to serve alongside the poultry, fish, or meat? Here are a few easy-to-prepare side dishes that will fit right in with the G.I. Diet.

- Green beans with almonds or mushrooms

- Mixed vegetables, such as sliced carrots, broccoli or cauliflower florets, and halved Brussels sprouts

- Boiled new potatoes (2 to 3 per serving), tossed with chopped herbs and a smidgen of olive oil

- Basmati rice. (You can stir some extra vegetables into the rice during the last few minutes of cooking.) Limit the serving size to 3 tablespoons uncooked rice, which will give you ⅔ of a cup when cooked, covering a quarter of the plate.

- Pasta—about 1¼ ounces uncooked, for ¾ cup cooked, covering a quarter of the plate

Meat

Veal and lean deli ham are your best choices. Red meat in general is a yellow-light food, although for pragmatic reasons, I've included lean cuts of beef and extra-lean ground beef in Phase I. Pork and lamb tend to have a higher fat content and should be avoided until Phase II. The serving size is critical. Remember, use the palm of your hand or a pack of playing cards as a guide to portion size. And please do not be alarmed by the apparent modest size of these servings. I had a real problem downsizing my steak at first, but now my stomach reels at the portions served in many restaurants.

---

steak dinner

For a complete steak dinner, try the following:

- Broil or grill fully trimmed lean beef steaks (4 ounces per person).

- Cook sliced onions and mushrooms with a little water in a nonstick skillet until softened. Use the onion and mushrooms to top the steak.

- Season asparagus, chopped broccoli, and halved Brussels sprouts with nutmeg and pepper, then microwave on high power until tender, 3 to 5 minutes. (Asparagus will cook the fastest; the Brussels sprouts will require more time).

- Boil 3 tablespoons uncooked basmati rice or two to three new potatoes per person. Season the cooked potatoes with chopped herbs and a touch of olive oil.

Meat Loaf

6 servings

1 ½ pounds extra-lean ground beef (less than 10 percent fat)
1 cup tomato juice
½ cup old-fashioned rolled oats
1 omega-3 egg, lightly beaten
½ cup chopped onion
1 tablespoon Worcestershire sauce
½ teaspoon salt (optional)
¼ teaspoon black pepper
Steamed vegetables and boiled small new potatoes, for serving

1. Preheat the oven to 350°F.

2. Place the beef, tomato juice, oats, egg, onion, Worcestershire sauce, salt, if using, and pepper in a large bowl. Mix lightly but thoroughly.

3. Press the meat loaf mixture into an 8-by-4-inch loaf pan.

4. Bake the meat loaf for about 1 hour, or until an instant-read meat thermometer inserted into the center registers 160°F.

5. Let the meat loaf stand for 5 minutes before draining off any juices and slicing it. Serve the meat loaf with a couple of vegetables and 2 to 3 small new potatoes.

Variation: Extra-lean ground beef is still relatively high in fat. A lower-fat and better alternative to ground beef is an equal amount of ground turkey or chicken breast. When fully cooked, ground turkey or chicken will register 170°F on an instant-read meat thermometer.

yogurt cheese

Looking for a green-light alternative to sour cream?
Try yogurt cheese—it's easy to make your own from
plain nonfat yogurt. Place a sieve lined with cheese-
cloth or paper towels on top of a bowl. Spoon the
yogurt into the sieve and cover it with plastic wrap.
Place the sieve and bowl in the refrigerator. Let the
yogurt drain overnight—the next day you'll have
yogurt cheese.

Chili

4 servings

2 teaspoons olive oil
1 large onion, sliced
2 cloves garlic, minced
½ pound extra-lean (less than 10 percent fat) ground beef
   or ground turkey (optional)
2 green bell peppers, chopped
2 cups canned tomatoes with juice
2 to 3 tablespoons chili powder
½ teaspoon cayenne pepper (optional)
½ teaspoon salt
½ teaspoon chopped fresh (or ¼ teaspoon dried) basil
2 cups water
1 can (19 ounces) red kidney beans, rinsed and drained
1 can (19 ounces) white kidney beans, rinsed and drained
Chopped tomato, chopped fresh parsley and cilantro, and/or yogurt
   cheese (see the box above) for garnish (optional).

1. Heat the olive oil in a deep skillet or saucepan over medium heat. Add the onion and garlic and sauté until nearly tender.

2. Add the ground meat, if using, and cook until browned, breaking up the chunks with a spoon. Drain off any fat.

3. Add the bell peppers, tomatoes, chili powder, cayenne, if using, salt, basil, and water and bring to a boil. Lower the heat and let simmer, uncovered, until the chili has reached the desired consistency, about 45 minutes.

4. Add the red and white kidney beans and cook over medium-low heat until heated through, about 5 minutes. Garnish the chili with tomato, parsley, cilantro, and/or yogurt cheese if desired. Serve.

SNACKS

Snacks play a critical role between meals, giving you a boost when you need it most. Have three a day: mid-morning, mid-afternoon, and before bed. Most popular snack foods are disastrous from a sugar and fat standpoint. Commercial cookies, muffins, and candy bars should be avoided at all costs. Fortunately, there are equally satisfying alternatives that are both convenient and low cost. Never leave home without them.

Here are a couple of recipes for between-meal pick-me-ups that won't weigh you down.

Apple Bran Muffins

Makes 12 muffins

Vegetable oil cooking spray
¾ cup wheat bran, such as All-Bran or Bran Buds
1 cup skim milk
⅔ cup whole wheat flour
Sweetener equivalent to ⅓ cup sugar
2 teaspoons baking powder
½ teaspoon baking soda
¼ teaspoon salt
1 teaspoon ground allspice
½ teaspoon ground cloves
1 ½ cups oat bran
⅔ cup raisins
1 large apple, peeled and cut into ¼-inch cubes
1 omega-3 egg, lightly beaten
2 teaspoons vegetable oil
½ cup applesauce (unsweetened)

1. Preheat the oven to 350°F. Spray a 12-cup muffin tin with vegetable oil cooking spray.

2. Mix the wheat bran and skim milk in a bowl and let stand for a few minutes.

3. In a large bowl, mix the flour, sweetener, baking powder, baking soda, salt, allspice, and cloves. Stir in the oat bran, raisins, and apple.

4. In a small bowl, combine the egg, oil, and applesauce. Stir, along with the wheat bran mixture, into the dry ingredients.

5. Spoon the batter into the prepared muffin tin. Bake until lightly browned, about 20 minutes. The muffins are done when a toothpick inserted in the center of one comes out clean. Keep the muffins in the freezer and microwave for 30 seconds on high power to warm.

---

snacking made simple

Want a green-light snack that requires no preparation on your part? Try one of these.

- 1 apple, pear, peach, or orange with a few almonds
- 4 ounces low-fat cottage cheese (1% or less) mixed with 1 teaspoon double-fruit, low-sugar preserves
- ¾ cup (6 ounces) fat-free fruit yogurt with sweetener
- ½ of a food bar such as Balance (200 calories, 20 to 30 grams carbohydrates, 12 to 15 grams protein, and 5 grams fat per bar)

Homemade Granola Bars

Makes 16 bars

1 ⅓ cups whole wheat flour
Sweetener equivalent to ⅓ cup sugar
2 teaspoons baking powder
¼ cup wheat bran, such as All-Bran or Bran Buds
1 teaspoon ground cinnamon
1 teaspoon ground allspice
½ teaspoon ground ginger
½ teaspoon salt (optional)
1 ½ cups old-fashioned rolled oats
1 cup finely chopped dried apricots
½ cup shelled sunflower seeds
¾ cup applesauce (unsweetened)
½ cup apple juice (unsweetened)
3 omega-3 eggs
2 teaspoons vegetable oil

1. Preheat the oven to 400°F.

2. Line a shallow 8-by-12-inch baking dish with parchment paper.

3. Mix the flour, sweetener, baking powder, wheat bran, cinnamon, allspice, ginger, and salt, if using, in a large bowl. Stir in the oats, apricots, and sunflower seeds.

4. Mix the applesauce, apple juice, eggs, and oil together, and add to the flour mixture.

5. Pour the batter into the prepared baking dish and spread it out evenly.

6. Bake until lightly browned, 15 to 20 minutes. Let cool and cut into 16 bars. Keep the bars in the freezer and microwave for 30 seconds on high power to warm.

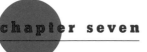

chapter seven

Phase II

Congratulations! You've achieved your new weight target!

Now is the moment to go back to page 26 and complete the chart you started a few months ago. Compare what you ate then with your current diet. I promise you'll be amazed at the change.

This may be hard to believe, but when I had reached my target weight—I had lost 22 pounds, and 3 inches off my waist—I had to make a conscious effort to eat more in order to avoid losing more weight. My wife said I was entering the "gaunt zone"!

PHASE II MEALS AND SNACKS

The objective in Phase II is to increase the number of calories you consume so that you maintain your new weight. Remember the equation: Food energy ingested must equal energy expended to keep weight stable. During Phase I, you were taking in less food energy than you were expending, using your fat reserves to make up the shortfall. Now we make up that deficit by taking in some extra food energy, or calories.

Two words of caution. First, your body has become accustomed to doing with fewer calories and has, to a certain extent, adapted. The result is that your body is more efficient than in the bad old days when it had more food energy than it could use. Second, your new lower weight requires fewer calories to function. For example, if you lost 10 percent of your previous weight, then you'll need 10 percent fewer calories for your body to function.

Combining a more efficient body, which requires less energy to operate, with a lower weight, which requires fewer calories, means that you need only a marginal increase in food energy to balance the energy in/energy out equation. The biggest mistake most people make when coming off a diet is assuming that they can now consume a much higher calorie level than their new body really needs. The bottom line is that Phase II is only marginally different from Phase I. Phase II provides you with an opportunity to make small adjustments to portion size and add new foods from the yellow-light category. All the fundamentals of the Phase I plan, however, remain inviolable. The following are some suggestions for how you might wish to modify your new eating pattern in Phase II:

Breakfast

- Increase cereal serving size, e.g., from ½ to ⅔ cup oatmeal.

- Add a slice of 100% whole-grain toast and a pat of margarine.

- Double up on the sliced almonds on cereals.

- Help yourself to an extra slice of Canadian bacon.

- Have a glass of juice now and then.

- Add one of the forbidden fruits—a banana or apricots—to your cereal.

- Have a fully caffeinated coffee. Try to limit yourself to one a day, and make sure it's a good one!

Lunch

I suggest you continue to eat lunch as you did in Phase I. This is the one meal that contained some compromises in the weight-loss portion of the program, since it is a meal most of us buy each day.

Dinner

- Add another boiled new potato (from two or three to three or four).
- Increase the rice or pasta serving from ¾ to 1 cup.
- Have a 6-ounce steak instead of your regular 4 ounce. Make this a special treat, not a habit.
- Eat a few more olives and nuts, but watch the serving size, as these are calorie heavyweights.
- Try a cob of sweet corn with a dab of nonhydrogenated margarine.
- Add a slice of whole-grain rye or pumpernickel bread.
- Have a lean cut of lamb or pork (maximum 4-ounce serving).

Snacks

Warning: Strictly watch quantity or serving size.

- Light microwave popcorn (maximum 2 cups)
- Nuts, maximum eight to ten
- A square or two of bittersweet chocolate (see below)
- A banana
- One scoop of low-fat ice cream or yogurt

Chocolate

To many of us, the idea of a chocolate-free world is abhorrent. The good news is that some chocolate, in limited quantities, is acceptable.

Most chocolate contains large quantities of saturated fat and sugar, making it quite fattening. However, chocolate with a high cocoa content (70 percent or more) delivers more chocolate satisfaction per ounce. So, a square or two of rich, dark, bittersweet chocolate, nibbled slowly or, better yet, dissolved in the mouth, gives us chocoholics just the fix we need. This high-cocoa chocolate is available at specialty stores and can even be found in some supermarkets.

Alcohol

Now is the moment that some of you have been waiting for. In Phase II, a daily glass of wine, preferably red and with dinner, is not only allowed—it's encouraged! Recently, there has been a flood of research into the benefits of alcohol on personal health. It is generally agreed that some alcohol is better than none at all, especially for heart health. It has been found that red wine in particular is rich in flavonoids and, when drunk in moderation (a glass a day), has a demonstrable benefit in reducing the risk of heart attack and stroke. The theory that says if one glass is good for you, two must be better is tempting but not true. One glass gives the optimum benefit.

As with coffee, if you're going to have only one glass of wine a day, make it a great one. My eldest son took me at my word about wine and gave me a subscription to the *Wine Spectator*. It has proven to be the most costly present I've ever received, as a whole new world of wine and wine ratings has opened up to me. My $10-a-bottle ceiling for special occasions has now doubled or tripled, though it has all been rationalized: I'm drinking less, so I can afford the extravagance!

As a beer aficionado, I like to drink the occasional beer as an alternative to wine. This habit has recently received an endorsement from a group of scientists, who reported in late 1999 that beer (in moderation) would reduce cholesterol and thus heart disease, delay menopause, and reduce the risk of several cancers. They also noted that beer has anti-inflammatory and anti-allergic properties, plus a positive effect on bone density. Personally, I worry about any product being touted as the wonder cure for all our ills, but clearly a glass of beer with supper is likely to do more good than harm.

But remember, because of its high malt content, beer is a high-G.I. beverage, so moderation is particularly important.

If you do drink alcohol, always have it with your meal. Food slows down the absorption of alcohol, thereby minimizing its impact.

THE WAY YOU WILL EAT FOR THE REST OF YOUR LIFE

With all these new options in Phase II, the temptation may be to overdo it. If the pounds start to reappear, simply revert to the Phase I plan for a while and you'll be astonished at how quickly your equilibrium is restored.

Phase II is the way you will eat for the rest of your life. You will look and feel better, have more energy, and experience none of those hypoglycemic lows. One reason, of course, that you have more energy is that you're not carrying around all that surplus fat. It might be fun to resurrect the backpack and load it up with the weight you've just lost. Carry it around on your back for an hour or two and then rejoice that you don't have to carry it around for the rest of your life! Whenever your resolve wavers, reach for the backpack. It's a marvelous motivator.

The opportunity to succeed is in your hands. I've tried to give you a simple yet motivating plan that will not leave you hungry, tired, or confused. It's all here in the book; the rest is up to you.

So, put on the backpack for a couple of hours, clear out the pantry, and drive to the supermarket. Remember to park as far as possible from the entrance and enjoy the extra walk. Everything starts with a first step!

LIVING WITH THE G.I. DIET

One of the most popular subjects in the many e-mail messages I receive is the practicality of "living with the G.I. Diet." Let me say from the outset, though I've designed the diet to be a realistic way to eat for the rest of your life, I don't expect anyone to adhere to it 100 percent of the time. Ninety percent would be a fair average. A good illustration is the reader who told me she was on the Vegas version of the G.I. Diet and had still lost 30 pounds. It appears that her version of the G.I. Diet was to allow herself one glass of red wine a day during Phase I (acceptable in Phase II but not in Phase I). She said that without that concession, she was really doubtful she would even have started the diet.

"Red days," as one of my cardiologist friends calls them, are inevitable in the real world, where dining out, family celebrations, holiday meals, business travel, and vacations all lend inevitably to some falling off the wagon.

Don't feel guilty when this occurs, as the worst that can happen is that it will take a little longer to realize your goals. Fortunately, one of the advantages of the G.I. Diet is the reaction of your body to red-light foods. After a few weeks of eating the G.I. Diet way, your body has become accustomed to low-G.I. foods that keep a steady sugar level in your blood. Enter a high-G.I. red-light food and immediately your sugar level zooms and a surge of insulin kicks in, leaving a surprised body fighting to regain its equilibrium!

Some people, like our glass-of-wine-a-day reader, find they can't live without certain products, peanut butter being another good example. If something is that important to you, by all means use it, but do so in strict moderation: for example, a 1-tablespoon serving of peanut butter per day. Otherwise, you're only kidding yourself, and risk overly slowing your progress.

We are all faced with inevitable situations where the menu is beyond our control: Thanksgiving, Christmas, weddings, business lunches or dinners. Here are a few suggestions on how you can minimize their impact on your program so that you can still enjoy the occasion and not appear to be a downer on others as well as yourself:

• Ask for extra vegetables in lieu of potatoes.

• Ask for salad dressing on the side so you control the quantity.

• Split a dessert with someone.

• Do not drink alcohol. In social situations, the pressure to drink "more than one" is very high and alcohol also tends to stimulate the appetite—a double whammy!

• Don't rush your food. The sooner you finish your food, the faster the opportunity and pressure for second helpings kick in.

• A removable travel and dining-out guide is available in Appendix IV for quick reference on what to eat when you have some control on the menu.

These rules are more relaxed in Phase II with the opportunity for larger serving sizes and the inclusion of yellow-light foods. Treat Phase II as part of your reward for achieving your goals in Phase I. Remember, this is how you are going to eat for the rest of your life. So don't view the G.I. Diet as a straitjacket. That is the certain road to disappointment.

Another guideline for living with the G.I. Diet is *moderation*. In order to keep the diet as simple as possible, I had to make certain assumptions as to how it would be interpreted. The basic assumption was that people would act in moderation and use their common sense. Because green-light products can in general be eaten in any quantity, I have assumed common sense would indicate that eating a jar of sugar-free applesauce or ten homemade granola bars at one sitting would not be acceptable. (Believe it or not, a couple of readers actually asked me about this.)

So common sense and moderation are key ingredients in living with the G.I. Diet and should always be borne in mind when assessing serving or portion sizes.

Finally, exercise. While exercise is not a key component in the relatively short time span of the weight-loss period in Phase I, it is an essential component in Phase II, the way you are going to eat and live for the rest of your life. For most people, simply walking thirty minutes a day (about 3 percent of your waking day) is quite sufficient. Get off the bus two stops early each way to work or park your car a mile from the office. That alone will burn up an extra pound of fat each month, giving you a little more flexibility in your diet as well as putting a spring in your step as you celebrate the new you.

---

to sum up

1. Don't treat the G.I. Diet as a straitjacket. Ninety percent compliance is an acceptable norm.

2. Use moderation and common sense in intepreting the diet, especially with serving and portion sizes.

3. Exercise, particularly walking, is an integral part of Phase II and the way you will eat and live for the rest of your life.

Let Me Hear From You I'm most interested in your feedback on the G.I. Diet. I would particularly like to hear about your personal experience with the diet and any suggestions you might be willing to share. Details are on my Web site, **www.gidiet.com.**

You will also find on the Web site the latest updates on the G.I. Diet, reader feedback, and sample recipes.

chapter eight

Exercise

Conventional wisdom has it that exercise is an essential component of a weight-loss program. Recent research findings strongly indicate that this is, in fact, *not* the case. Though any increase in an individual's level of activity is bound to burn up more calories, the net impact over the relatively short weight-loss period (typically twelve to twenty-four weeks) in Phase I is small.

Dieting will have a far greater impact on weight loss than exercise. To give you some idea of how much exercise is required to lose just one pound of weight, look at the following table:

EFFORT REQUIRED TO LOSE 1 POUND OF FAT

	130-POUND PERSON	160-POUND PERSON
Walking (4 mph–brisk)	53 miles/85 km	42 miles/67 km
Running (8-minute mile)	36 miles/58 km	29 miles/46 km
Cycling (12–14 mph)	96 miles/154 km	79 miles/126 km
Sex (average effort)	79 times	64 times

However, over the long haul, to maintain your new weight and for your overall health (especially heart health), exercise is an important contributor. For example, if you were to walk briskly for half an hour a day, seven days per week, you would burn up calories equaling 20 pounds of fat per year. *This means that in Phase I, exercise is not essential to your weight-loss program, but it is an important consideration in Phase II, where you maintain your new weight.*

Exercise has been an important part of my life since the age of thirty-eight, when I was humbled by my seven-year-old son. He challenged me to a run around the block—and he won soundly. I recognize that exercise is a subject many people don't want to hear about. Nevertheless, before you skip it totally, read the box below. If you still aren't convinced that you should read on, then this chapter is not for you.

---

regular exercise will:

1. assist in weight maintenance

2. dramatically reduce your risk of heart disease, stroke, diabetes, and osteoporosis

3. improve your mental well-being and boost your self-esteem

4. help you sleep better

For those couch potatoes who have been driven by curiosity to read this far, stay with me, and see if the following objections to regular exercise sound like your own: "It's painful," "It's boring," "I don't have the time." I am going to address all three complaints head-on.

First, let's look at the pain or discomfort excuse. This probably comes from an experience where you tried to do too much too soon. The world's basements are full of exercise equipment purchased in a moment of excessive enthusiasm—probably coupled with some

New Year's resolutions. A few weeks later, aching muscles, a sore bottom, and burning lungs have relegated that exercise bike or other, more exotic machine to the deep, dark storeroom where we put things that "may be useful later." Sound familiar?

To avoid pain, you must start small and work yourself up. Ten years ago, I was an active jogger, running twenty-five to thirty miles a week. Unfortunately, I developed a back disc problem (totally unrelated to jogging) and it was nine years before I ventured out again. After winning my personal battle of the bulge, I couldn't believe the problems that my re-entry to jogging created. Day one saw me enthusiastically bounding out the door in my beautiful new running shoes. Half a mile later, I stopped in a wheezing heap, lungs burning, knees aching, calf muscles in spasm. You're probably thinking, "Serves him right," confirming for yourself that exercise is a painful option.

The reason I'm relating this story is that I had to learn the hard way. Jogging is a wonderful exercise, but it places a high demand on your body, particularly if you're over forty. Since I fell into that age category, I had to find an alternative exercise that required less physical effort and was more in tune with the realities of my aging body. I decided to start walking. If you start small and work yourself up, it is a pain-free exercise (see page 110).

The second objection to exercise is boredom. I am very sympathetic to this one. While some exercises, such as jogging, walking, and bicycling, are rarely boring because they take place outdoors, for some of us, winters can be a disincentive. The nine years I spent working out on my exercise bike and ski machine in the basement were more of a challenge. Granted, this wasn't my only option. Many people use fitness clubs for both the motivation ("I've paid my fee, so I'd better use it") and the social interaction and mutual encouragement. One or two of the well-heeled have personal trainers, but this is unrealistic for most of us.

Instead, I chose the basement, as there was no fitness facility nearby. My solution to the inherent boredom came via an ancient

TV abandoned by the children as they left the nest, and an early "play only" VCR. I recorded those shows and films that ran between midnight and six A.M. on the family VCR, and they provided my entertainment. I pedaled and skied my way through James Bond movies, build-your-own-cottage shows, and Jacques Cousteau undersea documentaries. There was never a boring moment. In fact, I sometimes became so engrossed in the shows that I exercised far beyond my scheduled time allocation. Indoors, a little ingenuity (which could be as simple as putting on a Walkman) can help make workouts more interesting.

The last objection is lack of time. There are 336 thirty-minute blocks of time each week. Take 2 percent of these blocks, just 7 blocks total, and use one each day. This can hardly be an unreasonable allocation of your time, especially when you consider the benefits: a slimmer, fitter, healthier you! Thirty minutes a day should be your target, though I know that many of you will want to increase this allocation once you feel the remarkable improvements that such a modest time commitment can bring.

As far as what time of day you should exercise is concerned, there are two camps: those who are at their best first thing in the morning and those who warm up during the day to hit their peak in the evening. I strongly suggest you align your exercise activity with whichever camp you fall into. In our household, I'm the morning person, who cannot imagine exercising at the end of the day as my watch spring winds down. My wife, conversely, dreads the mornings but is a force to be reckoned with by the time we get home in the evening. Needless to say, we don't exercise together. So choose your best time—either bounding out of bed to greet the dawn or exercising away accumulated tensions at the end of the day. Either way, exercise will be an enjoyable component of your daily routine.

Many people find that as their level of fitness increases, they sleep better and wake up feeling more refreshed, taking less time to drag themselves from bed. This in itself frees up more time for exercise, resulting in even less of a draw upon your day.

When referring to "exercise," I am talking about aerobic, or cardio, exercise, which boosts the heart rate and causes you to breathe harder. But before we look at the options and getting started, let's talk further about exercise.

WEIGHT LOSS AND MAINTENANCE

One thing we need to get straight right off: Exercise is *not* a substitute for dieting. Dieting will have a far greater impact on weight loss than exercise. What brought home this point to me was the annual rowing race between Oxford and Cambridge Universities on the Thames. Rowing, along with water polo, is rated as the toughest physical endurance test for the body because it uses every muscle we have, and the race is more than four miles long. It amazed me to find out that each rower consumed the calorie equivalent of only one bar of chocolate during the race! Obviously, an enormous expenditure of energy is needed to offset our poor dietary habits. But exercise is an essential complement to diet. Together, the two will give you optimum weight loss and, even more important, maintain your new healthy weight.

Exercise works in exactly the same way as diet to reduce or control weight. The more energy (calories) you expend than you take in, the more your body will use up your energy reserve (fat) to make up the shortfall. Exercise burns calories. In fact, every action you perform uses calories. So, climbing the stairs instead of taking the elevator to your office, getting off the bus a stop or two early, or parking as far away as possible from the mall or supermarket entrance will require extra activity over your normal routine and thereby consume extra calories.

As I noted earlier, if you were to walk briskly for half an hour a day while continuing to eat a good regular diet, you would lose 20 pounds a year automatically. How come? Well, a brisk half-hour walk consumes approximately 200 extra calories. Multiply that by

365 days and you get 73,000 calories, or 20 pounds (1 pound = 3,600 calories).

(*Note:* The thirty-minute (1½ miles) walk that burns 200 calories is based on a 150-pound person. Heavier people will burn more calories in thirty minutes, and lighter people will burn fewer. A 200-pound person will burn 220 calories, a 130-pound person 175 calories. And the more briskly you walk, the more calories you will consume.)

Exercise has two further benefits on weight loss and control. First, exercise increases your metabolism—the rate at which you burn up calories—*even after you've finished exercising.* In other words, the benefits stay with you all day. Exercise in the morning is particularly beneficial as it sets the pace for your metabolism for the day.

A second bonus is that exercise builds muscle mass. Starting at the age of twenty-five, the body loses 1.5 percent of its muscle mass each year. High-protein, low-carbohydrate diets accelerate that loss. By exercising muscles on a regular basis, the loss can be minimized or reversed. And why is that important? Because the larger your muscles, the more energy (calories) they use. When you're at rest, or even asleep in bed, your muscles are using energy. So keeping or building muscle mass really helps you to burn calories and lose weight.

Though regular exercise will help minimize muscle loss, it is resistance exercises that actually build muscle mass. Resistance exercises are those where weights, elastic bands, or hydraulics are used for muscles to pull or push against. Most of you are probably cringing at the thought of sweating bodybuilders doing endless painful workouts with massive barbells and other daunting equipment. As I will show a little later, though, it does not have to be like that. A few simple exercises will do wonders to tone and restore those flabby muscles.

We will deal with the other health benefits of exercise in chapter 9 when we look at the impact of weight on your health, in particular on heart disease and stroke, which accounts in North America for four deaths out of every ten.

GETTING STARTED

Even if you are not thrilled at the prospect of exercise, it's important to get started. Here are some ways to make it more appealing to you.

1. Select an exercise that suits you. The fastest way to abandon an exercise program is to do something you don't enjoy. It is best to select an exercise that uses the largest muscle groups, that is, the legs, abdominals, and lower back. These muscles burn more calories because of their sheer size. Walking, jogging, and biking are excellent choices.

2. Get support from family and friends. If possible, find a like-minded buddy so you have support and motivation.

3. Set goals and keep a record. A removable exercise log (see page 153) is included to help keep you on track. Put it on the fridge or in the bathroom.

4. Make sure your doctor supports your plan.

   Now let's review your options.

OUTDOOR ACTIVITIES

Walking

This is by far the simplest and, for most people, the easiest exercise program to start and maintain. Thirty minutes a day, seven days a week, should be your target. If you add an hour-long walk on the weekend, you can take a day off during the week. As mentioned before, we're talking about brisk walking—not speed walking or ambling. It must increase your heart and breathing rates, but never exercise to the point where you cannot find the breath to converse with a partner.

You don't need any special clothing or equipment except a pair of comfortable cushioned shoes or sneakers. And walking is rarely boring, since you can keep changing routes and watch the world go by as you exercise. Walk with a friend for company and mutual support, or go solo and commune with nature and your own thoughts. I do my best thinking of the day on my morning walk. This is not surprising when you realize how much extra oxygen-fresh blood is pumping through your brain.

A great idea is to incorporate your walking into your daily commute to work. I get off the bus three stops early on my way to and from work. Those three stops are equal to about 1½ miles, so I'm walking about 3 miles per day! If you drive to work, try parking your car about 1½ miles away and walk to your job. You may even find cheaper parking farther out.

Jogging

This exercise is similar to walking, but more care is needed with footwear to protect joints from damage. The advantage of jogging over walking is that it approximately doubles the number of calories burned in the same period of time—400 calories for jogging versus 200 for brisk walking over a thirty-minute period. While walking, try jogging for a few yards and see if this is for you. It will get your heart rate up, which is great for heart health. The heart is basically a muscle, and, like all muscles, it thrives on being exercised—in general, the more the better. If jogging is for you, then this could arguably be the simplest and most effective method of exercise, as it uses personal time efficiently, can be done anytime, anywhere, and is inexpensive.

Hiking

Another version of walking is cross-country hiking. Because this usually involves varying terrain, especially hills and valleys, you use up more calories—about 50 percent more than for brisk walking. The reason is that you use considerably more energy going uphill, as your body literally has to lift its own weight from the bottom to the top. Try hauling 150 to 200 pounds up a hill and you'll get some idea of the extra effort your body has to make. Hiking is a great deal of fun, too, especially on weekends when you can get out of town. It also provides a change of pace from your regular walking or jogging routine.

Bicycling

Like walking, jogging, and hiking, bicycling is a fun way to burn up calories, and it is almost as effective as jogging. Again, other than the cost of the bike, it's inexpensive and can be done almost anywhere and anytime. It can also be done indoors during winter months in colder climates with a stationary bike.

Bicycling offers another good change of pace from your regular routine. I find it gives me a chance to visit all sorts of communities outside my normal walking range.

Other Outdoor Activities

In-line skating, ice-skating, skiing (especially cross-country), snowshoeing, and swimming (in a lake or pool) are good alternatives to or changes of pace from any of the above activities. They are similar to biking in terms of energy consumption.

Sports

Though most sports are terrific calorie burners, they usually cannot be part of a regular routine. Most require other people, equipment, and facilities, all of which mitigate against a continuing, regular exercise program. But, again, they can be an excellent top-off or boost to your regular fitness and exercise program. Popular sports such as tennis, basketball, soccer, softball, and golf (no golf cart, please) are excellent adjuncts to a basic exercise program. But they are not a substitute for a five-to-seven-day-a-week regular schedule.

Indoor Activities

Many of you will be muttering by now about how this would all sound fine if we lived in California, but many of us have either frigid, snowy winters or hot, humid summers to contend with, making outdoor activities unattractive.

The alternative is either a home gym or a fitness club. The latter is an easy option these days in most larger communities. Clubs offer not only a wide range of sophisticated equipment, but also mutual support from friends and expert advice from staff.

If a fitness club isn't convenient or those Lycra-clad young things make you uncomfortable, the simple alternative is to exercise at home. The best and least expensive piece of equipment is a stationary exercise bike. The latest models work on magnetic resistance rather than the old friction strap around the flywheel. This gives a smoother action with better tension adjustment. Most important, they are quiet, which is crucial if you want to be able to listen to music or watch TV.

You can easily pay into the thousands for a bike with all the fancy trimmings, one that is designed for use in a fitness club, but in reality the $200 to $300 machine will work fine. Just be sure it has smooth, adjustable tension and seat height, then pop in that late-night movie or your favorite soap and get pedaling. You'll be amazed how quickly the minutes fly by. Twenty minutes on the bike will give you the same calorie consumption as thirty minutes of brisk walking.

If biking is not for you, try a treadmill. These can be expensive, and beware of the lower-end models that cannot take the pounding. Expect to pay about $600 to $900, and make sure that the incline of the track can be raised and lowered for a better workout.

Both treadmills and bikes can simulate outdoor walking, jogging, hiking, or biking in the comfort of your own home. I use both of these machines but have added a cross-country ski machine, which has the advantage of working the upper body as well. Ski machines are generally less expensive than treadmills but cost more than stationary bikes. They also burn a considerably higher number of calories (similar to jogging) because they use the arms and shoulders as well as the legs—almost the perfect all-body workout machine.

There are several other more specialized options, such as stair-step and rowing machines, but they are not for everyone. They are also quite expensive, so make sure you try them out first at a fitness club or with a cooperative retailer.

---

note

Most authorities support the notion that any extra activity is better than none at all. I have no argument with that, but experience shows that if people start substituting washing the car or throwing the ball with the dog as alternatives to a regular brisk exercise program, then the program does not work. By all means garden, wash the windows, or do whatever else you like, but please do not fool yourself into thinking that this will have a significant impact on your weight loss or maintenance program.

Resistance Training

It's now time to pay some attention to rebuilding your muscle mass. Remember that after age forty, you will lose between 4 and 6 pounds of muscle every decade, which is usually replaced with flab. That's 4 to 6 pounds of calorie-consuming muscle. Muscles burn up energy even when idle. Let me illustrate this point with an analogy. As a student, I pumped gas during one of my vacations.

One day a pre-war Bentley drove in and the owner asked me to fill it right to the top. He left the car running and went to the washroom. The car was filled through a large pipe that stuck about eighteen inches out of the gas tank. I was not able to fill the tank to the top of the pipe because the level kept dropping with every beat of the huge twelve-cylinder engine. I had to ask the owner to switch off the engine so I could finally top it off! The point is that, like the Bentley, bigger muscles consume more energy than smaller muscles, even when idling.

Resistance-training equipment can range from the complex and expensive to the simple and inexpensive. Home gyms are a popular option for a few hundred dollars and up. For most people, however, there are much simpler methods—free weights or (my own preference) rubber bands. Dynaband and Thera-Band are two popular choices. The latter I find particularly useful, as it comes in varying thicknesses, offering increasing levels of resistance as you regain and build your muscle strength.

Thera-Band comes in rolls of six-inch-wide rubber strips, in different colors for different thicknesses (the thicker the band, the more resistance to stretching). The big advantage of this form of resistance training is that it's inexpensive ($10 to $20), so lightweight that you can take it anywhere, and progressive, providing a psychological boost as you trade up to the next level of resistance (there are eight levels). You'll find a list of suggested exercises in Appendix VI.

After two years of use, I've now reached the maximum resistance level with Thera-Band, so I've added some 5-pound wrist and ankle weights to the workout. These resistance rubber bands and weights are available at many fitness exercise equipment retailiers and surgical supply stores.

Try a few resistance exercises, concentrating on the larger muscle groups—your legs, arms, and upper chest. These are the muscles that will give you the biggest bang by burning up the most calories. The resistance exercises should add to your other regular exercise regimen, not replace it. Muscle-building exercise is strictly complementary to regular get-your-body-moving exercise. Using both types of exercise together will work far better than either one alone. And resistance exercises are best done every other day, leaving time for your muscles to recuperate.

For a complete exercise overview, including instructions for warm-up, strengthening, and stretching exercises, see Appendix VI.

---

to sum up

1. A regular exercise program will accelerate weight loss and help you maintain a desired weight. It will also improve your health (especially heart health), help you feel good, and allow you to sleep better. It will be the best thirty-minute-a-day investment you'll ever make.

2. Choose an activity that suits your personality and your schedule.

3. Stick to it. Make it part of your life at least five days a week—preferably every day.

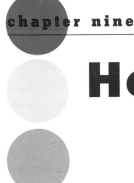

chapter nine

Health

Foods are, in effect, drugs. They have a powerful influence on our health, well-being, and emotional state. We take in food four or five times a day, usually with more thought for taste than for nutritional value. It would be incomprehensible to take drugs on the same basis.

The right foods can help you maintain your health, extend your life span, give you more energy, and make you feel good and sleep better. Couple that with exercise and you are doing all you can to keep healthy, fit, and alert. The rest is a matter of genes and luck.

Let's take a quick look at the importance of diet and exercise in preventing diseases.

HEART DISEASE AND STROKE

Given that I was the president of the Heart and Stroke Foundation of Ontario for fifteen years, it is hardly surprising that I'm starting with a discussion of these diseases. However, there is a more important reason: Heart disease and stroke cause 40 percent of North American deaths. Remarkably, this is evidence of progress. When I first joined the foundation, the figure was close to 50 percent.

This is a good news, bad news story. The good news is that advances in surgery, drug therapies, and emergency services have saved many lives. The bad news is that twice as many deaths could have been averted if only we had reduced our weight, exercised regularly, and quit smoking. Though the smoking rate for adults has dropped sharply (unfortunately, we cannot say the same for teens), we are eating more and exercising less, leading inevitably to a more obese and unhealthy population. It's been calculated that if we led even a moderate lifestyle, we could halve the carnage from these diseases. Though heart disease, like most cancers, is primarily a disease of old age, nearly half of those who suffer heart attacks are under the age of sixty-five.

A familiar refrain that I have heard many times is, "Why worry? If I have a heart attack, modern medicine will save me." It might well save you from immediate death, but what most people do not realize is that the heart is permanently damaged after an attack. The heart cannot repair itself because its cells do not reproduce. (Ever wonder why you cannot get cancer of the heart? That's the reason.) After the damage sustained during a heart attack, the heart has to work harder to compensate—but it rarely can. It slowly degenerates under this stress, and patients finally "drown" as blood circulation fails and the lungs fill with liquid. Congestive heart failure is a dreadful way to die, so make sure you do everything you can to avoid having a heart attack in the first place.

With regard to diet, the simple fact is that the fatter you are, the more likely it is you will suffer a heart attack or stroke. The two key factors that link heart disease and stroke to diet are cholesterol and hypertension (high blood pressure). I promised at the beginning of this book that I was not going to dwell on the complexities of the science of nutrition; it's the outcome of this science that's important. However, a little science is helpful to understand the role and importance of both hypertension and cholesterol.

Hypertension, or high blood pressure, is the harbinger of both heart disease and stroke. High blood pressure puts more stress on the arterial system and causes it to age and deteriorate more rapidly, ultimately leading to arterial damage, blood clots, and heart attack or stroke. Excess weight has a major bearing on high blood pressure. A Canadian study in 1997 found that obese adults, aged eighteen to fifty-five, had a five- to thirteen-times greater risk of hypertension. A further study demonstrated that a lower-fat diet coupled with a major increase in fruits and vegetables (eight to ten servings a day) lowered blood pressure. The moral: Lose weight and eat more fruits and vegetables to help reduce your blood pressure levels. In other words, adopt the G.I. Diet.

Cholesterol is essential to your body's metabolism. However, high cholesterol is a problem, as it's the key ingredient in the plaque that can build up in your arteries, eventually cutting off the blood supply to your heart (causing heart attack) or your brain (leading to stroke). To make things more complicated, there are two forms of cholesterol: HDL (good) cholesterol and LDL (bad) cholesterol. The idea is to boost the HDL level while depressing the LDL level. (Remember it this way: HDL is Heart's Delight Level and LDL is Leads to Death Level.)

The villain that raises LDL levels is saturated fat, which is usually solid at room temperature and is found primarily in meat and whole milk and certain food products. Conversely, polyunsaturated and monounsaturated fats not only lower LDL levels but actually boost HDL. The moral: Make sure some fat is included in your diet, but make sure it's the right fat. (Refer to chapter 1 for the complete rundown on fat.)

DIABETES

Diabetes is the kissing cousin of heart disease, in the sense that more people die from heart complications arising from diabetes than from diabetes alone. And diabetes rates are skyrocketing: They are expected to double in the next ten years.

The principal causes of the most common form of diabetes, Type 2, are obesity and lack of exercise, and the current epidemic is strongly correlated to the obesity trend. The most dramatic illustration of this link appears in North America's native population, where in some communities diabetes affects nearly half the adult population. Before the Europeans colonized North America, the native peoples lived in a state of feast or famine. When there was an abundance of food, plant or animal, it was stored in the body as fat. In lean times, such as winter, the body depleted these fat supplies. As a result, their bodies developed a "thrift gene," with those who stored and utilized their food most effectively being the survivors—a classic Darwinian exercise in survival of the fittest. When you take away the need to hunt or to harvest food—that is, the need to exercise—and replace it with a trip to the supermarket whenever food is required, the result is inevitable: a massive increase in obesity and, with it, diabetes.

Foods with a low-G.I., which release sugar more slowly into the bloodstream, appear to play a major role in helping diabetics control their disease. Thus the G.I. Diet provides an opportunity both to lose weight and to assist in the management of the disease. Prevention, however, is far preferable, so get right into your G.I. Diet program and exercise plan, and get those pounds off.

CANCER

The connection between diet and cancer is less distinct. However, a recent global report by the American Institute for Cancer Research concluded that 30 to 40 percent of cancers are directly linked to dietary choices. Its key recommendation is that individuals should choose a predominantly plant-based diet that includes a variety of vegetables, fruits, and grains—the G.I. Diet in a nutshell.

chapter ten

Supplements

As a young advertising account executive in the United Kingdom, I was briefed by a nutritionist on vitamin supplements that Miles Labs was planning to introduce into England. The nutritionist was skeptical about the readiness of the British for these American-style multivitamin therapies and whether people even needed them. Her comment—"Our sewers contain the richest concentration of vitamins in the country"—still resounds in my head whenever the question of vitamins and other food supplements comes up.

There is a great deal of truth in what she said. Most of us get at least the minimum recommended levels of most vitamins and minerals from our diet. There is increasing evidence, however, that the usual RDA (Recommended Daily Allowance) may be insufficient in certain specific instances. This is a dynamic area of nutrition research and very susceptible to change as new data pours in on a daily basis. Based on our present knowledge, here are some guidelines that may be helpful.

Vitamin B

Vitamin B, especially B_6, B_{12}, and folic acid, is critical to good health. Principal sources of vitamin B are seafood and meat. It is important to note that excessive amounts of some B vitamins can be harmful.

There is growing evidence that vitamin B is a key ingredient in combating a chemical called homocysteine, which attacks your arteries. This substance can be triggered by digesting excessive amounts of animal protein. This again suggests that high-protein diets can be dangerous to your health by not only stimulating the production of homocysteine but also generating unacceptable levels of vitamin B.

The levels in most one-a-day multivitamins (20 mcg B_{12}, 2 mg B_6, 400 mcg folic acid) are quite sufficient to make up for any possible deficiencies in your diet.

Vitamin C

This is certainly the most popular vitamin sold, mainly because of its association with cold prevention and reduction. Though there is little evidence to support that traditional claim, we do know that vitamin C is critical to muscles, ligaments, and joints.

While the G.I. Diet, with its emphasis on fresh fruit and vegetables, will certainly cover your basic vitamin C requirements, topping off with a one-a-day multivitamin may help.

Vitamin D

This is the true sunshine vitamin, and not vitamin C, as the Florida ads suggest. Though vitamin D is prevalent in milk and fatty fish, our body can produce vitamin D itself only when exposed to sunshine. For those of us in more northern climes, sunshine is a scarce commodity in winter, and since we should be lathered in sunscreen during the summer (protecting the skin but inhibiting vitamin D production), we are unable to capitalize on this vitamin self-generation.

Vitamin D is important because it facilitates the processing of calcium for your bones. This is critical for people over fifty, especially women, in order to prevent osteoporosis. A shortage of vitamin D can also bring on aches and pains similar to symptoms of arthritis.

Again, the G.I. Diet, with its emphasis on low-fat dairy and fish, will help, but it won't hurt to supplement with a multivitamin, which normally contains the recommended daily level of 400 IU.

Vitamin E

This became the wonder vitamin of the 1990s when it was suggested that it could reduce the chance of developing heart disease, Alzheimer's, and certain cancers. There are many significant population studies currently under way, though recent heart disease reports have questioned its benefit.

Vitamin E is the one principal vitamin that is underrepresented in most multivitamins. The recommended daily dosage is 100 to 400 IU, whereas most multivitamins contain only 30 to 50 IU. The G.I. Diet will give you a good natural supply of vitamin E, which is found in vegetable oils and nuts (both also sources of "good" fat). However, you would require a significant intake of these vegetable fats to realize the recommended levels. Taking a 400 IU vitamin E supplement is therefore a good idea and carries little risk.

Fish Oil

There is one oil in particular that has been found to have significant positive health benefits, especially for your heart. The oil is called omega-3, and it is a fatty acid found primarily in coldwater fish, salmon in particular, as well as in canola and flaxseed. As most of us are unlikely to consume salmon on a daily basis (or enough canola or flaxseed), salmon oil is available in capsule form in any pharmacy. I take a couple at breakfast (2,000 mg) every day. The research evidence supporting omega-3 is overwhelming and much of it stems from studies of the Inuit, who do not eat what we consider a heart-healthy diet; theirs is loaded with animal fat and lacks pretty much any fruits or vegetables. However, the coldwater fish they consume, rich in omega-3, appear to give them protection against heart disease.

to sum up

The G.I. Diet almost certainly contains sufficient vitamins to meet your daily needs. However, if you are at all concerned, a one-a-day multivitamin offers cheap and risk-free insurance. An extra vitamin E pill is optional, but keep your ears and eyes open to new research on this front. If heart health is a particular concern, omega-3 oil capsules are a good idea.

The Complete G.I. Diet Food Guide

	RED LIGHT	YELLOW LIGHT	GREEN LIGHT
beans	Baked beans with pork Refried beans	Kidney beans (canned) Lentils (canned)	Baked beans (canned)* Black-eyed peas Chickpeas Kidney beans Lentils Lima beans Navy beans Peas Pinto beans Soybeans Split peas
beverages	Alcoholic drinks (in general) Regular soft drinks	Beer** Coffee (with skim milk, no sugar) Diet soft drinks (caffeinated)	Bottled water Club soda Decaffeinated coffee (with skim milk, no sugar)

*Limit quantity.

**In Phase II, a glass of wine and an occasional beer may be included. Red wine in moderation has been shown to have cardiovascular benefits.

	● RED LIGHT	● YELLOW LIGHT	● GREEN LIGHT
beverages (continued)		Fruit juices (unsweetened) (see page 33) Wine (preferably red)*	Diet soft drinks (no caffeine) Tea (with skim milk, no sugar)
breads	Bagels Baguette/ Croissants Cake/Cookies Cornbread English muffins Hamburger buns Hot dog buns Kaiser rolls Melba toast Muffins/ Doughnuts Pancakes/ Waffles Pizza Regular granola bars Stuffing Tortillas White bread	Pita bread (whole wheat) Sourdough bread Tortillas (low-carb) Whole grain breads	Homemade Apple Bran Muffins (page 93) Homemade Granola Bars (page 95) 100% stone-ground whole wheat bread** Whole-grain, high fiber bread**

*In Phase II, a glass of wine and an occasional beer may be included. Red wine in moderation has been shown to have cardiovascular benefits.

**Use a single slice only per serving; 2½–3 grams fiber per slice.

	RED LIGHT	YELLOW LIGHT	GREEN LIGHT
cereal grains	Millet Rice (short grain, white, instant) Rice cakes	Corn	Barley Buckwheat Bulgur Rice (basmati, brown, long grain, wild) Wheat berries
cereals	All cold cereals except those listed as yellow or green light Cream of Wheat Granola Grits Muesli (commercial) Instant/Quick-cook oatmeal	Post Shredded Wheat 'N Bran	All-Bran Bran Buds Fiber One Homemade Muesli (see page 72) Kashi Go Lean Large-flake oatmeal (e.g., Quaker Old-Fashioned Oats) Oat bran
condiments/ seasonings	Croutons Ketchup Mayonnaise Tartar sauce	Mayonnaise (light)	Garlic Herbs/Spices Hummus Mayonnaise (fat-free) Mustard Soy sauce (low sodium) Teriyaki sauce Vinegar Worcestershire sauce

	● RED LIGHT	○ YELLOW LIGHT	● GREEN LIGHT
dairy	Cheese Chocolate milk Cottage cheese (whole or 2%) Cream Cream cheese Ice cream Milk (whole or 2%) Sour cream Yogurt (whole or 2%)	Cheese (low-fat) Cream cheese (light) Ice cream (low-fat) Milk (1%) Sour cream (light) Yogurt (low-fat with sugar)	Buttermilk Cheese (fat-free) Cottage cheese (1% or fat-free) Cream cheese (nonfat) Ice cream* (low-fat and no added sugar) Milk (skim) Frozen Yogurt (nonfat and no added sugar) Fruit Yogurt (nonfat and sugar-free) Sour cream (fat-free) Soy/whey protein powder
fats/oils	Butter Coconut oil Hard margarine Lard Mayonnaise Palm oil Peanut butter Salad dressings (regular) Tropical oils Vegetable shortening	Corn oil Mayonnaise (light) Most nuts Peanut oil Salad dressings (light) Sesame oil Soft margarine (nonhydrogenated) Sunflower oil Vegetable oil	Almonds* Canola oil*/seed Flaxseed Hazelnuts* Macadamia nuts* Mayonnaise (fat-free) Olive oil* Salad dressings (fat-free) Soft margarine* (nonhydrogenated, light; e.g., Promise Ultra) Vegetable oil sprays

*Limit quantity (see page 56).

	🔴 RED LIGHT	🟡 YELLOW LIGHT	🟢 GREEN LIGHT
fruits (fresh)	Cantaloupe Dates Honeydew melon Melons Prunes Raisins* Watermelon	Apricots Bananas Kiwis Mangoes Papayas Pineapple	Apples Blackberries Blueberries Cherries Grapefruit Grapes Lemons Oranges (all varieties) Peaches Plums Pears Raspberries Strawberries
fruits (bottled, canned, frozen)	All canned fruit in syrup All dried fruit* Applesauce containing sugar	Apricots Fruit cocktail in juice	Applesauce (unsweetened) Frozen berries Mandarin oranges Peaches/pears in juice or water
fruit juices**	All fruit drinks All sweetened juices Prune Sorbet Watermelon	Apple (unsweetened) Cranberry (unsweetened) Grapefruit (unsweetened) Orange (unsweetened) Pear (unsweetened) Pineapple (unsweetened)	

*For baking, it is okay to use a modest amount of dried fruits.

**Whenever possible, eat the fruit rather than drink its juice.

	● RED LIGHT	● YELLOW LIGHT	● GREEN LIGHT
meat/ poultry/ fish/eggs	Bologna Bratwurst Ground beef (more than 20% fat) Regular eggs Hamburgers Hot dogs Pastrami Processed meats Regular bacon Salami Sausages Sushi rolls	Ground beef (lean—10–20% fat) Omega-3 eggs Lamb (lean cuts) Pork (lean cuts) Regular eggs Turkey bacon	All seafood, fresh, frozen, or canned (in water)* Beef (lean cuts) Canadian bacon Chicken breast (skinless) Liquid eggs Egg Beaters Egg whites Ground beef (extra lean—less than 10% fat) Lean deli ham Sashimi Smoked salmon Tofu Turkey breast (skinless) Veal
pasta**	All canned pastas Couscous Gnocchi Macaroni and cheese Noodles (canned or instant) Pasta filled with cheese or meat		Capellini Fettuccine Linguine Macaroni Penne Spaghetti Vermicelli
pasta sauces	Alfredo sauces with added meat or cheese Sauces with added sugar or sucrose	Sauces with vegetables	Light sauces with vegetables (no added sugar); e.g., Colavita and Classico

*Avoid breaded or coated seafood.

**Use whole wheat or protein-enriched pastas if available.

	● RED LIGHT	● YELLOW LIGHT	● GREEN LIGHT
snacks	Bagels Bread Candy Cookies Crackers Doughnuts French fries Ice cream Jell-O Muffins (commercial) Popcorn (regular) Potato chips Pretzels Raisins Rice cakes Tortilla chips Trail mix	Bananas Dark chocolate** (70% cocoa) Ice cream (low-fat) Most nuts Popcorn (light, microwavable)	Almonds* Applesauce (unsweetened) Canned peaches/ pears in juice or water Cottage cheese (1% or fat-free) Food bars*** Frozen yogurt (nonfat and no added sugar) Fruit Yogurt (non-fat and no added sugar) Hazelnuts* Homemade Apple Bran Muffins (page 93) Homemade Granola Bars (page 95) Ice cream (low-fat and no added sugar) Macadamia nuts* Most fresh fruit (see page 129) Most fresh veg-etables (see page 132)
soups	All cream-based soups Black bean Green/split pea Pureed vegetable Chicken noodle Lentil	Tomato	Chunky bean and vegetable soups (e.g., Campbell's Healthy Request and Healthy Choice)

*Limit quantity (see page 56).

**For chocoholics only; high cocoa (70%) dark chocolate *in small quantities*. Treat as a concession and eat only occasionally.

***180- to 225-calorie bars, e.g., Balance; ½ bar per serving.

	RED LIGHT	YELLOW LIGHT	GREEN LIGHT
sugar and sweeteners	Corn syrup Glucose Honey Molasses Sugar (all types)	Fructose	Aspartame Equal Splenda Sugar Twin Sweet'N Low
vegetables	French fries Hash browns Parsnips Potatoes Potatoes (instant, mashed, or baked) Rutabagas Turnips	Artichokes Beets Corn Potatoes (boiled) Pumpkin Squash Sweet potatoes Yams Asparagus Avocado* Beans (green/wax) Bell peppers Broccoli Brussels sprouts Cabbage Carrots Cauliflower Celery	Collard greens Cucumbers Eggplant Leeks Lettuce (all varieties) Mushrooms Okra Olives* Onions Peas Peppers (hot) Pickles Potatoes (boiled new)** Radishes Snow peas Spinach Tomatoes Zucchini

*Limit quantity (see page 56).

**2 to 3 served whole or sliced (not mashed) per serving in Phase I; 3 to 4 in Phase II.

Green-Light Kitchen Cupboard Essentials

PANTRY

baking/cooking

Sliced almonds
Dried apricots
Baking powder/soda
Cocoa (70%)
Wheat/oat bran
Whole wheat flour

beans (canned)

Baked beans (low-fat)
Mixed salad beans
Soybeans
Vegetarian chili

breads

100% stone-ground
whole wheat

cereals

All-Bran
Bran Buds
Fiber One
Kashi Go Lean
Oatmeal (large flake)

drinks

Bottled water
Club soda
Decaffeinated
coffee/tea
Milk (skim)
Diet decaffeinated
soft drinks

fats/oils

Canola oil
Margarine
(soft, light)
Mayonnaise (nonfat)
Olive oil
Salad dressings
(nonfat)
Vegetable oil sprays

fruit
(canned/bottled)

Applesauce
(unsweetened)
Mandarin oranges
Peaches in juice or water
Pears in juice or water

pasta (whole wheat)

Fettuccine
Spaghetti
Vermicelli

pasta sauces
(vegetable-based
only)

Classico
Colavita

rice

Basmati, brown, long
grain, wild

seasonings

Flavored vinegars/
sauces
Spices/herbs

snacks

Food bars (Balance)

**soups (vegetable-
or bean-based
only)**

Healthy Choice
Healthy Request

sweeteners

Equal
Splenda
Sugar Twin
Sweet'N Low

vegetables

Potatoes (new, small
only)
Tomatoes

FRIDGE

dairy

Buttermilk
Cottage cheese (1%)
Milk (skim)
Fruit yogurt (fat- and
sugar-free)

fruit

Apples
Blackberries

Blueberries
Cherries
Grapefruit
Grapes
Lemons
Limes
Oranges
Peaches
Pears
Plums
Raspberries
Strawberries

**meat/poultry/
fish/eggs**

Ground beef (extra
lean)
Chicken breast (skin-
less)
Egg Beaters
Egg whites
Ham/turkey/chicken
(lean deli)
Liquid eggs
Seafood, fresh, frozen,
or canned in water (no
batter or breading)
Turkey breast
(skinless)
Veal

vegetables

Asparagus
Beans (green or wax)
Bell peppers
Broccoli
Cabbage
Carrots
Cauliflower
Celery

Cucumber
Eggplant
Leek
Lettuce
Mushrooms
Olives
Onion
Peppers (hot)
Pickles
Radishes
Snow peas
Spinach
Zucchini

FREEZER

dairy

Ice cream (nonfat and
no sugar added)
Frozen yogurt (nonfat
and no sugar added)

snacks

Apple Bran Muffins
(page 93)
Homemade Granola
Bars (page 95)

vegetables/fruit

Mixed berries
Mixed peppers
Mixed vegetables
Peas

G.I. Diet Shopping List

PANTRY

baking/cooking

- [ ] Baking powder/ soda
- [ ] Cocoa (70%)
- [ ] Dried apricots
- [ ] Sliced almonds
- [ ] Wheat/oat bran
- [ ] Whole wheat flour

beans (canned)

- [ ] Baked beans (low-fat)
- [ ] Most varieties
- [ ] Mixed salad beans
- [ ] Vegetarian chili

bread

- [ ] 100% stone-ground whole wheat

cereals

- [ ] All-Bran
- [ ] Bran Buds
- [ ] Fiber One

- [ ] Kashi Go Lean
- [ ] Oatmeal (large flake)
- [ ] Soy protein powder

drinks

- [ ] Bottled water
- [ ] Club soda
- [ ] Decaffeinated coffee/ tea
- [ ] Diet decaffeinated soft drinks

fats/oils

- [ ] Canola oil
- [ ] Margarine (soft, light)
- [ ] Mayonnaise (nonfat)
- [ ] Olive oil
- [ ] Salad dressings (nonfat)
- [ ] Vegetable oil spray

fruit (canned/bottled)

- [ ] Applesauce (unsweetened)

- [ ] Mandarin oranges
- [ ] Peaches in juice or water
- [ ] Pears in juice or water

pasta

- [ ] Capellini
- [ ] Fettuccine
- [ ] Macaroni
- [ ] Penne
- [ ] Spaghetti
- [ ] Vermicelli

pasta sauces (vegetable-based only)

- [ ] Classico
- [ ] Colavita

rice

- [ ] Basmati
- [ ] Brown
- [ ] Long grain
- [ ] Wild

seasonings

☐ Flavored
vinegars/sauces

_____

_____

_____

_____

☐ Spices/herbs

_____

_____

_____

_____

_____

snacks

☐ Food bars (Balance)

soups

☐ Healthy Choice
☐ Healthy Request

sweeteners

☐ Equal, Splenda,
Sugar Twin, Sweet'N
Low (and other non-
sugar sweeteners)

FRIDGE/ FREEZER

dairy

☐ Buttermilk
☐ Cottage cheese (1%)
☐ Frozen yogurt
(nonfat and no sugar
added)
☐ Fruit-based yogurt
(fat- and sugar-free)
☐ Ice cream (low-fat
and no sugar added)
☐ Milk (skim)
☐ Sour cream (nonfat)

fruit

☐ Apples
☐ Blackberries
☐ Blueberries
☐ Cherries
☐ Grapefruit
☐ Grapes
☐ Lemons
☐ Limes
☐ Oranges
☐ Peaches
☐ Pears
☐ Plums
☐ Raspberries
☐ Strawberries

meat/poultry/ fish/eggs

☐ Chicken breast
(skinless)
☐ Egg Beaters

☐ Egg whites
☐ Ground beef (extra
lean)
☐ Ham/turkey/chicken
(lean deli)
☐ Liquid eggs
☐ Seafood, fresh,
frozen, or canned in
water (no batter or
breading)
☐ Turkey breast
(skinless)
☐ Veal

vegetables

☐ Asparagus
☐ Beans (green/wax)
☐ Bell and hot peppers
☐ Broccoli
☐ Cabbage
☐ Carrots
☐ Cauliflower
☐ Celery
☐ Cucumber
☐ Eggplant
☐ Leeks
☐ Lettuce
☐ Mushrooms
☐ Olives
☐ Onions
☐ Pickles
☐ Potatoes (new, small
only)
☐ Snow peas
☐ Spinach
☐ Tomatoes
☐ Zucchini

appendix IV

Dining Out
and Travel Tips

	● RED LIGHT	● GREEN LIGHT
breakfast	Bacon/Sausage Bagels Cold cereals Eggs Muffins Pancakes/Waffles	All-Bran Egg whites/Egg Beaters— Omelet (no cheese, please) Egg whites/Egg Beaters— Scrambled Fruit Oatmeal Yogurt (nonfat, no sugar added)
lunch	Bakery products Butter/Mayonnaise Cheese Fast food Pasta-based meals Pizza/Bread/Bagels Potatoes (replace with double vegetables)	Meats—deli ham, chicken, or turkey breast Pasta—¼ plate maximum Salads—low-fat (dressing on the side) Sandwiches—open-face, whole wheat Soups—chunky vegetable and bean Vegetables Wraps—½ pita or low-carb tortilla, no mayonnaise

	● RED LIGHT	● GREEN LIGHT
dinner	Beef/Lamb/Pork Bread Butter/Mayonnaise Caesar salad Desserts—pastries, ice cream, candy Pasta-based meals Potatoes (replace with double vegetables) Soups—cream based White rice (regular)	Chicken/turkey (no skin) Fruit Pasta—¼ plate Rice (basmati, brown, long grain, wild)—¼ plate Salads—low-fat (dressing on the side) Seafood—not breaded or battered Soups—chunky vegetable or bean Vegetables
snacks	Candy Chips (all types) Cookies/Muffins Popcorn (regular) Pretzels	Fresh fruit Light cottage cheese with unsweetened fruit preserves Nuts (preferably almonds, hazelnuts, or macadamia nuts, 8–10) Yogurt—nonfat, no sugar ½ Food bar (e.g., Balance)

PORTIONS

Meat/Fish	Palm of hand/Pack of cards
Vegetables	Minimum ½ plate
Rice/Pasta	Maximum ¼ plate
New potatoes	2 to 3 in Phase I; 3 to 4 in Phase II

Exercise Calorie Counter

CALORIES BURNED PER 30 MINUTES OF EXERCISE

Weight (in Pounds):	130	160	200
Gym and home activities			
Aerobics: low-impact	172	211	264
Aerobics: high-impact	218	269	336
Aerobics, step: low-impact	218	269	336
Aerobics, step: high-impact	312	384	480
Aerobics, water	125	154	192
Bicycling, stationary: moderate	218	269	336
Bicycling, stationary: vigorous	328	403	504
Circuit training: moderate	250	307	384
Rowing, stationary: moderate	218	269	336
Rowing, stationary: vigorous	265	326	408
Ski machine: moderate	296	365	456
Stair step machine: moderate	187	230	288
Weight lifting: moderate	94	115	144
Weight lifting: vigorous	187	230	288

CALORIES BURNED PER 30 MINUTES OF EXERCISE

Weight (in Pounds):	130	160	200
Training Activities			
Basketball: playing a game	250	307	384
Basketball: wheelchair	203	250	312
Bicycling: BMX or mountain	265	326	408
Bicycling: 12–13.9 mph	250	307	384
Bicycling: 14–15.9 mph	312	384	480
Boxing: sparring	281	346	432
Football: competitive	281	346	432
Football: touch, flag, general	250	307	384
Frisbee	94	115	144
Golf: carrying clubs	172	211	264
Golf: using cart	109	134	168
Gymnastics	125	154	192
Handball	374	461	576
Hiking: cross-country	187	230	288
Horseback riding	125	154	192
Ice-skating	218	269	336
In-line skating	218	269	336
Martial arts	312	384	480
Racquetball: casual, moderate	218	269	336
Racquetball: competitive	312	384	480
Rock climbing: ascending	343	422	528
Rock climbing: rappelling	250	307	384
Rope jumping	312	384	480
Running: 5 mph (12 min/mile)	250	307	384
Running: 5.2 mph (11.5 min/mile)	281	346	432

CALORIES BURNED PER 30 MINUTES OF EXERCISE

Weight (in Pounds):	130	160	200
Running: 6 mph (10 min/mile)	312	384	480
Running: 6.7 mph (9 min/mile)	343	422	528
Running: 7.5 mph (8 min/mile)	390	480	600
Running: 8.6 mph (7 min/mile)	452	557	696
Running: 10 mph (6 min/mile)	515	634	792
Running: pushing wheelchair, exercise stroller	250	307	384
Running: cross-country	281	346	432
Skiing: cross-country	250	307	384
Skiing: downhill	187	230	288
Snowshoeing	250	307	384
Softball	156	192	240
Swimming	187	230	288
Tennis	218	269	336
Volleyball: noncompetitive, general play	94	115	144
Volleyball: competitive, gymnasium play	125	154	192
Volleyball: beach	250	307	384
Walking: 3.5 mph (17 min/mile)	125	154	192
Walking: 4 mph (15 min/mile)	140	173	216
Walking: 4.5 mph (13 min/mile)	156	192	240
Walking/Jogging: jogging more than 10 min	187	230	288
Water polo	312	384	480
Waterskiing	187	230	288
White-water rafting, kayaking	156	192	240

CALORIES BURNED PER 30 MINUTES OF EXERCISE

Weight (in Pounds):	130	160	200
Daily Life Activities			
Children's games: 4-square, etc.	156	192	240
Chopping and splitting wood	187	230	288
Gardening	140	173	216
Housecleaning	109	134	168
Mowing lawn: push, hand	172	211	264
Operating snow blower: walking	140	173	216
Raking lawn	125	154	192
Sex	47	58	72
Shoveling snow: by hand	187	230	288

Strengthening & Resistance Exercises

Overview

In order to minimize the risk of injury and maximize the impact of exercise, my physiotherapist recommends exercising in the following order:

1. Warm-up
2. Targeted stretching
3. Aerobic/cardiovascular workout activity
4. Strengthening
5. Stretching/cool-down

Warm-up

Warming up is not stretching. Stretching cold muscles can damage them. Warm-ups are procedures to raise your body temperature in preparation for exercise. Methods can vary from a hot shower or sauna to just doing the activity at a slower pace.

Targeted Stretching

I recommend specific stretching before a workout only if you have a specific requirement dut to an injury such as a lower-back injury. You may therefore need to do exercises that have been prescribed by your health practitioner prior to the workout activity.

Aerobic/Cardiovascular Workout Activity

Aerobic/cardiovascular exercise will burn calories and increase your overall health, especially your heart's health. Detailed information is available in chapter 8.

Strengthening

I recommend that strengthening be done after the aerobic/cardiovascular activity, when your body is warm and ready for the intensity of the exercise. Strengthening exercises should be done on alternate days to allow muscles time to recover. Having two alternating strength programs works well for many people. For example, one day you can do your arm workout and the next day your legs. This also reduces the length of time for each workout. The only strengthening exercises recommended on a daily basis are those for the trunk muscles, i.e., the muscles that support your mid and lower spine. It seems that these generally do better if they are worked every day.

The number of strengthening repetitions is determined by your goals. For most of us, the goal is to maintain or build muscle mass, to be toned, and to have the endurance to do everyday activities with less effort. To achieve these goals, start at a weight or resistance (Thera-Band) level where you can perform fifteen repetitions without feeling overly fatigued on completion. You should repeat this set of exercises two or three times in a session, with a minute rest between each set. You can use the rest time effectively by exercising a different set of muscles and then performing the second or third set later in the workout.

The biggest mistake most people make is increasing their weights or resistance too quickly. This frequently results in an injury and an inability to exercise for several weeks or even months. Many of us make the decision to increase the demands of the program based on the length of time we have been doing the exercise. We assume that because we have been exercising regularly, we must eventually make the program more difficult. This is a false assumption. Though it is true that, as we are growing and peaking physically, we can generally increase the demands on our body, it is not the same once we have peaked. Most people hit their physical peak around age thirty-five. If you are in your mid-thirties or older, do not look at your exercise program as one that should get progressively harder, longer, or more demanding once established.

How do you know when you are ready to increase the weights or resistance? If you are able to do fifteen repetitions comfortably, I recommend increasing the repetitions to gain what I term a "margin for error." Take the repetitions up in groups of five until you can do thirty. Once you can comfortably do thirty repetitions, then go to the next level of resistance or weight and drop back down to fifteen repetitions. Continue to use this pattern to increase the difficulty of your program as you feel ready.

It is okay to do the same workout for a prolonged period of time. You may want to choose different exercises to prevent boredom, but the program does not have to get harder or more time-consuming for you to continue to benefit.

An excellent book on weight training is *Strength Training Past 50*, by Wayne Westcott and Thomas Baechle. Though it is geared to the fifty-plus age group, it is ideal for anyone.

Strengthening Exercises

Abdominal

1. Lying on your back on the floor, tighten your stomach muscles without moving your back or pelvis. Your back should be held still throughout this exercise. Your stomach will be flat or concave. Your arms are on the floor by your side.

2. Feel the contraction with your fingertips, and maintain this position throughout the next stage.

3. Lift one leg to a bent hip and knee position so your thigh is vertical and your calf is parallel to the floor.

4. Bring the second leg up beside it. This must be achieved without your back moving.

5. Slowly straighten one leg horizontally to the floor. Do not allow it to touch the floor.

6. Straighten the knee fully or to the point where you feel you may lose the stomach contraction, then return to the starting position.

7. Repeat fifteen times with each leg, two to three sets.

Hips and Knees

1. Stand on a stair step or a 4- to 6-inch-high stool.

2. Slowly bend one leg, lowering the other foot *almost* to the floor. If balance is a problem, slide your back against the wall—if on the stairs, hold on to banister.

3. Repeat fifteen times with each leg, two to three sets.

4. Progress by increasing the height of the stool.

Legs and Buttocks

This exercise is a variation on the traditional "going up on your toes." You should concentrate on slowly lifting your heels off the ground by squeezing your buttocks as well as using your calf muscles. Imagine you are in a vertical shaft and must go straight up the shaft rather than move forward onto your toes. This uses more muscles as well as larger ones.

Hold for two to three seconds. Repeat five times, two to three sets.

Thera-Band
Strengthening Exercises

Diagonal Trunk Strengthening

1. Stand with your feet shoulder width apart.

2. Place the Thera-Band under your feet. Keep your knees slightly bent.

3. Holding the Thera-Band in one hand, pull the band from your hip to over the opposite shoulder. Do not let your trunk twist. Keep your elbows straight.

4. Repeat fifteen times on each side, two to three sets.

Biceps

1. Place a single band under one foot. Hold the band in the hand on the same side, arms at rest.

2. Bend your elbow to touch your hand to your shoulder. Keep your wrist straight.

3. Repeat fifteen times with each arm, two to three sets.

Triceps

1. Place your right hand against your chest.

2. Put your left hand against the right.

3. Grasp the Thera-Band in both hands.

4. Pull the left hand straight out from the chest. The closer together the two hands are on the Thera-Band, the more difficult the exercise.

5. Repeat fifteen times with each arm, two to three sets.

Ws

1. With your hands at your shoulders (elbows raised to a 90-degree angle) and the Thera-Band behind your neck, pull out to a 45-degree angle.

2. Repeat fifteen times, two to three sets.

You may progress with these exercises by doubling the band before going to the next level of resistance.

Caution: Elastic resistance should not be continued to maximum fatigue.

Hips and Knees

Resisted Hip Abduction

1. With one end of the Thera-Band around your leg and the opposite end secured in a door jamb, stand sideways from the door and extend your leg out to the side, 18 to 24 inches.

2. Repeat fifteen times with each leg, two to three sets.

Resisted Hip Extension

1. With one end of the Thera-Band around your leg and the opposite end secured in a door jamb, face the door and pull your leg straight back.

2. Repeat fifteen times with each leg, two to three sets.

Note: To lengthen the life of your Thera-Band, take a piece of nylon webbing (2 feet) and tie it in a loop. Thread and knot the Thera-Band through the loop. Webbing loop and knot are then secured between the door jamb and the door.

For additional information and other Thera-Band strengthening exercises, visit www.theraband.com.

Stretching/Cool-Down

You should stretch at the end of your exercise program for a couple of reasons. It's calming, helping you to "come down" from the intensity of your workout, and it lengthens your muscles after they've been shortened and tightened while exercising. The ideal time to stretch is when the body is warmed up, following a workout or perhaps even in the shower. The length of time you should hold stretches varies from ten seconds to one minute, but I recommend holding each stretch for one minute. There is a wide range of books and brochures readily available on stretching exercises, or you could check the Internet.

Some people complain that no matter how much they stretch, they never get more flexible. These people are called "musclebound." They're usually strong and even flexible—but in the wrong areas. For example, someone may have an extremely tight hamstring muscle, which is at the back of the thigh. To compensate for the leg tightness, he or she may have increased flexibility in the lower back. People with this type of flexibility often look like a question mark when they try to stretch their hamstring muscles. Without being aware of it, they are stretching their back until it's extremely rounded. Very little of the force they're exerting is going into lengthening the muscle they're trying to stretch. If this sounds like you, ask a health practitioner who understands compensatory muscle patterns to show you how to prevent your body from "cheating." It is very important to learn correct stretching techniques, particularly if you have poor flexibility or if you have a lower back or neck problem. It is also essential to have good trunk strength to prevent any compensatory patterns.

The Ten Golden G.I. Diet Rules

1. Eat three meals and three snacks every day. Don't skip meals—particularly breakfast.

2. In Phase I, stick with green-light products only.

3. When it comes to food, quantity is as important as quality. Shrink your usual portions, particularly of meat, pasta, and rice.

4. Always ensure that each meal contains the appropriate measure of carbohydrates, protein, and fat.

5. Eat at least three times more vegetables and fruit than usual.

6. Drink plenty of fluids, preferably water.

7. Exercise for thirty minutes once a day or fifteen minutes twice a day. Get off the bus/subway two stops early or park your car a mile from your destination.

8. Find a friend to join you for mutual support.

9. Set realistic goals. Try to lose an average of a pound a week and record your progress to reinforce your sense of achievement.

10. Don't view this as a diet. It's the basis of how you will eat for the rest of your life.

G.I. DIET WEEKLY WEIGHT/WAIST LOG

week	date	weight	waist	comments
1.				
2.				
3.				
4.				
5.				
6.				
7.				
8.				
9.				
10				
11.				
12.				
13.				
14.				
15.				
16.				
17.				
18.				
19.				
20.				

G.I. DIET EXERCISE LOG T=time D=distance

date	walking	jogging	bicycling	resistance (repetitions)	stretching	other
T						
D						
T						
D						
T						
D						
T						
D						
T						
D						
T						
D						
T						
D						
T						
D						
T						
D						
T						
D						
T						
D						
T						
D						
T						
D						
T						
D						
T						
D						

Index

To determine whether a specific food is green-light, yellow-light, or red-light, please refer to Appendix I: The Complete G.I. Diet Food Guide (pages 125–132).

A

abdominal exercises, 146
abdominal fat, 17
aerobic exercise, 108
Agriculture Department, U.S., 7
    Food Pyramid of, 27, *28*
alcohol:
    in Phase I, 55
    in Phase II, 99–100
American Heart Association, xi
American Institute for Cancer
        Research, 120
animal protein, 14
antioxidants, in tea, 54
apple bran muffins, 93–94
apples, as green-light food, 64
Asian stir-fry, 84
Atkins, Robert C., xii
Atkins diet, xii

B

bacon, 35
barley, as green-light food, 64
baseline measurements, 59
beans, 125
    as green-light food, 64–65
    as protein source, 14
beer, 99–100
beverages, 125–26
    in Phase I, 52–55
biceps, strengthening of, 147
bicycling, 112
blood sugar, 101

alcohol consumption and, 55
    Glycemic Index and, 10–12, *10, 11*
BMI, *see* body mass index
body fat:
    BMI and, 16
    effort to lose one pound of, 104
    energy stored in, 17, 20
    glucose and, 11
    measurement of, 17, *18–19*
    pound-per-week loss of, 22
body mass index (BMI), 16–17,
        18–19
    serving sizes and, 57
body shape, 17
brain food, 15
bran, 7
    in apple muffins, 93–94
    in cold cereal, 73
    as green-light food, 66–67
breads, 126
    as green-light food, 65
    in Phase I breakfast, 31, 34
    in Phase I dinner, 47
    in Phase I lunch, 37, 39
breakfast:
    meal ideas, 71–76
    on-the-run, 74
    in Phase I, 30–35
    in Phase II, 97
burgers, fast food, 40
butter, *5*

C

caffeine, 53–54
calories:
    average adult need for, 20
    burned in exercise, 108–9, 139–42
    on food labels, 60, 61
    reduction of, 21–23

in traditional vs. G.I. diet, *21*
cancer, diet and, 120
canned fruit, as green-light food, 67
canola oil, 4–5, *5*, 70, 123
carbohydrates, xii, 6–9
  in food pyramids, *28*
  in Phase I breakfast, 31–32
  in Phase I dinner, 47–48
  in Phase I lunch, 37–38
  restriction of, xii
cardiovascular exercise, 108
cereal, cold, 73
cereals, 127
  as green-light food, 65
  in Phase I breakfast, 31, 33
cheese, 71
  yogurt, 69
chicken:
  basic preparation of, 83
  curry, 86
  fast-food, 40
  Italian, 85
  and rice salad, 80
chili, 91–92
Chinese food, 41
chocolate, in Phase II, 98–99
cholesterol:
  alcohol and, 99
  cardiovascular disease and, 118
  fiber and, 9
  HDL and LDL forms of, 119
  saturated fats and, 4
cocoa content, in chocolate, 99
coconut oil, 4
coffee, 35, 53–54
coldwater fish, omega-3 and, 5,
  123–24
color-coded categories, *30–32*
condiments, 127
  in Phase I lunch, 38
cooling down, 149–50
corn oil, *5*
cottage cheese:
  and fruit, 82
  as green-light food, 65
curried chicken, 86

D
daily life activities, calories burned in,
  142
dairy, 128
  in Phase I breakfast, 30, 33–34
  in Phase I dinner, 47
  in Phase I lunch, 36
  as protein source, 14
  vitamin D in, 122
dessert, in Phase I, 43, 52
diabetes, xiii–xiv, 119–20
  glucose and, xiv
  heart disease and, xiv
  Type 2, 17, 120
diet, cancer and, 120
diets (weight loss):
  food-specific, xi
  high-protein, xii
digestion, foods processed in, 12–13
dining out, G.I. Diet and, 137–38
dinner:
  meal ideas, 83–92
  in Phase I, 30–35, 36–43, 46–52
  in Phase II, 98
dressings, for salads, 78
Dynaband, 115

E
eggs, 130
  as green-light food, 65
  in omelets, 74–76
  in Phase I, 43
  in Phase I breakfast, 30, 34
  in Phase I dinner, 46–47
  in Phase I lunch, 36
  scrambled, 76
elastic bands, 109, 115
electrolytes, xii
energy:
  from carbohydrates, 6
  from fat, 17, 20
  food processed into, 3
  from glucose, 10–12
equipment, resistance-training, 115
exercise, xi, 103, 104–16
  calories burned in, 108–9, 139–42

choosing time of day for, 107
getting started in, 110
machines for, 113–14
sleep improved by, 107
sports as adjunct to, 112
time allotted to, 107
Type 2 diabetes and, 120
weight loss and maintenance with,
108–10
see also resistance training
exercise log, 153

F
fad diets, xi–xii
fast food, 39–41, 55
fat, body, see body fat
fats, dietary, 3–6, 5, 70–71, 128
cholesterol levels and, 119
digestion of, 13
and energy, 3
on food labels, 60, 61
in food pyramids, 28
in oils, 4–5
in Phase I breakfast, 32
in Phase I dinner, 49
in Phase I lunch, 38
saturated, 4
fiber, 9, 34
in beans, 14
digestion of, 13
on food labels, 60, 61
fish, 41, 130
basic preparation of, 87
as green-light food, 68–69
as omega-3 source, 5, 50, 123–24
in Phase I dinner, 49–50
as protein source, 14
vitamin D in, 122
fish oil, 5, 123–24
flavonoids, 99
flaxseed oil, 5, 123
flour, white, 7
folic acid, 122
Food and Drug Administration
(FDA), 27
food guide, for G.I. diet, 125–32

food journal, template for, 26
Food Pyramid:
G.I. Diet, 28, 29
U.S.D.A., 6–7, 27, 28
food ratios, in G.I. diet, 20–21, 21, 29
food-specific diets, xi
free weights, 115
fries, fast food, 40
fruit drinks, in Phase I, 54–55
fruits, 129
in Phase I breakfast, 31, 33
in Phase I dinner, 48
in Phase I lunch, 37–38

G
G.I. Diet:
color-coded categories in, 29,
30–32
dining out and travel tips for,
137–38
food guide of, 125–32
food ratios in, 20–21, 21
"living with," 101–3
Phase II of, 23, 96–100
Phase I of, 21–23, 25–57
shopping list for, 135–36
special occasions and, 101–2
ten golden rules of, 151
weekly logs for, 152–53
glossary, of green-light foods, 64–69
glucose, xiii–xiv
from carbohydrates, 6
energy from, 10–12
fat storage and, 11
Glycemic Index, xiii–xiv, 9
description of, 10–13
ratings and charts of, 10, 11
grains, 6–8, 8, 127
in food pyramids, 27, 28
in Phase I breakfast, 31
in Phase I dinner, 47
in Phase I lunch, 37
granola bars, homemade, 95
grapefruit, as green-light food, 66
green-light foods, 64–69, 125–32
described, 23

glossary, 64–69
kitchen cupboard essentials in,
    133–34
in Phase I breakfast, 30–32
in Phase I dinner, 46–49
in Phase I lunch, 36–39
in Phase I snacks, 45
serving sizes of, 56
side dishes as, 88
snacks as, 94
gym activities, calories burned in, 139

H
hamburgers, as green-light food, 66
Harvard School of Public Health, 21
HDL cholesterol, 119
Healthy Weight Pyramid, of Mayo
    Clinic, 27, 29
heart, heart disease, 13
    alcohol and, 99
    diabetes and, xiv
    fats and, 4–5
    statistics on, 109, 117
    weight and, 117–19
Heart and Stroke Foundation of
    Ontario, xi, xiii, 117
high blood pressure, 118–19
high-G.I. foods, 10–13, *10*, 62
high-protein diets, xii, 14, 109
hiking, 111–12
hip and knee exercises, 146, 148–49
holidays, G.I. diet and, 101–2
home exercises, calories burned in, 139
homemade granola bars, 95
homemade muesli, 72
hydrogenated oils, 4
hyperglycemia, xiv
hypertension, 118–19
hypoglycemia, 62

I
ice cream, as green-light food, 66
indoor exercising, 113–14
insoluble fiber, 9
instant foods, 8
insulin production:

alcohol and, 55
caffeine and, 53
fat storage and, 11, 12
high-G.I. foods and, 11, 12, 62,
    101
sugar consumption and, 11
Inuits, diet of, 123–24
Italian chicken, 85
Italian omelet, 75

J
Jenkins, David, xiii–xiv
jogging, 106, 111
juices, 129
in Phase I, 54–55
in Phase I breakfast, 22, 32

K
ketosis, xii

L
labels, Nutrition Facts and, 60–61
LDL cholesterol, 119
leg and buttocks exercises, 147
legumes, as green-light food, 64–65
low-fat proteins, 14
low-G.I. foods, 12–13, 20, 27, 101
lunch:
    meal ideas, 77–82
    in Phase I, 30–35, 36–43
    in Phase II, 98

M
machines, for exercise, 113–14
margarine, soft, 5
Mayo Clinic, Healthy Weight
    Pyramid of, 27, 29
meal ideas, 70–95
meat loaf, 90
meats, 89–92, 130
    in Phase I breakfast, 30, 35
    in Phase I dinner, 46–47, 49–50
    in Phase I lunch, 36
    as protein source, 14
    substitutes for, 50–51
Mediterranean diet, 5

metabolism, 109
Metropolitan Life, 16
Mexican food, 41
Mexican omelet, 75
Miles Labs, 121
milk, as green-light food, 66
milk shakes, 40
milling, of grains, 7–8, 65
moderation, 99, 101, 102
monounsaturated fats, 4–5, 14–15,
      119
motivation, 62
muesli, 71, 72
muffins, apple bran, 93–94
multivitamins, 122–23
muscle mass, 109, 114–16

N
nutrition bars, as green-light food, 66
Nutrition Facts, on food labels,
      60–61
nuts:
      as green-light food, 66–67
      as protein source, 14–15

O
oat bran, *see* bran
oatmeal, 8–9, 71–72
      as green-light food, 65, 67
      in homemade granola bars, 95
obesity, 120
      on BMI index, *18–19*
      as pervasive problem, 2, *2*
oils (cooking), *5*, 70, 128
      fats in, 4–5
      hydrogenated, 4
      partially hydrogenated, 4
olive oil, 4–5, *5*, 70
omega-3, 50, 65, 123–24
omelets, 74–76
on-the-run breakfast, 74
oranges, as green-light food, 67
outdoor activities, 110–12
overweight:
      on BMI index, *18–19*
      in Western hemisphere, 2, *2*

P
palm oil, 4
pantry items, getting set and, 59–60
partially hydrogenated oils, 4
pasta, 130
      as green-light food, 67
      in Phase I, 42
      in Phase I dinner, 51
      salad, 80–81
      U.S. consumption of, 7
peaches, as green-light food, 67
peanut butter, 101
pears, as green-light food, 67
Phase I, 21–23, 25–57
      beverages in, 52–55
      breakfast in, 30–35
      dinner in, 46–52
      food journal for, 26
      and food pyramids, 28
      lunch in, 36–43
      portions and, 27, 29, *29*
      serving sizes in, 55–57
      snacks in, 44–45
Phase II, 23, 96–100
      alcohol in, 99–100
      as lifelong program, 100
      meals and snacks in, 96–99
pizza, 41
plaque, 119
polyunsaturated fats, 4, 119
potatoes, 132
      as green-light food, 68
      in Phase I dinner, 51
      in Phase I lunch, 42–43
poultry, 83–86, 130
      basic preparation of, 83
      as protein source, 14
prepared foods, 8–9
preserves, in Phase I breakfast, 34
processed foods, 7–8
protein, 13–15
      animal, 14
      as "brain food," 15
      digestion of, 13
      in food pyramids, 28
      harmful amounts of, xii, 14

in Phase I breakfast, 30
in Phase I dinner, 46–47
in Phase I lunch, 36
sources of, 14–15

R
recipes, *see* meal ideas
Recommended Daily Allowance
    (RDA), 121
"red days," 101
red-light foods, 101, 125–32
    described, 22
    in Phase I breakfast, 30–32
    in Phase I dinner, 46–49
    in Phase I lunch, 36–39
    in Phase I snacks, 45
resistance training, 109, 114–16, 143–50
    muscles developed by, 114–16
rice:
    and chicken salad, 80
    as green-light food, 68–69
    in Phase I dinner, 51
    in Phase I lunch, 43
root vegetables, 132
    as green-light food, 68
rowing, 108
rubber bands, 109, 115

S
salad, in Phase I dinner, 48, 51–52
salade niçoise, 79
salads, 77–81
    fast-food, 40
    variations on, 78
salmon oil, 123
sandwiches, 81
sashimi, 68
saturated fats, xii, 4
sauces, 130
scrambled eggs, 76
seafood:
    in Phase I dinner, 49–50
    as protein source, 14
Sears, Barry, xiii
seasonings, 127
serving sizes, 55–57

on food labels, 60, 61
shellfish, 41
shopping, getting set with, 60
side dishes, green-light, 88
skim milk, in Phase I, 53
slow-release foods, xiv, 9, 120
snacks, 7, 93–95, 131
    hydrogenated oils in, 4
    meal ideas, 93–95
    in Phase I, 44–45
    in Phase II, 98
soft drinks, in Phase I, 53
soft margarine, 5
soluble fiber, 9
Sonnenblick, Edmund H., ix
soups, 131
    as green-light food, 68
    in Phase I dinner, 49
    in Phase I lunch, 39, 42
soy-based products, 50–51
sports:
    calories burned in, 140–41
    as exercise adjuncts, 112
spreads, in Phase I breakfast, 34
steak dinner, 89
stir-fry, Asian, 84
strengthening exercises, 143–50
stretching, 143, 149–50
stroke, 109, 117–19
    alcohol and, 99
submarines (sandwiches), 41
sugar:
    avoidance of, 27
    glycemic index and, 10–12, *10, 11*
sugar substitutes, *see* sweeteners
sunflower oil, 5
sushi, as green-light food, 68–69
sweeteners, 27, 73, 132
    as green-light food, 69

T
tea, 35
    in Phase I, 54
Thera-Band, 115, 147–49
"These Nine Products Are Killing
    Americans," 4

"thrift gene," 120
tofu, 50–51
    as green-light food, 69
trans fatty acids, 4
travel, 137–38
triceps, strengthening of, 148
tropical oils, 4
trunk strengthening, 147
turkey breast, basic preparation of, 83
Type 2 diabetes, 17, 120

U
United Kingdom, 121
United States:
    fat consumption in, 6
    food recommendations of, 27
    grain consumption in, 6–8, *8*
    overweight in, 2, *2*
    pasta consumption of, 7
USDA, *see* Agriculture Department,
    U.S.

V
vegetable protein, 14–15
vegetables, 132
    in Phase I breakfast, 32
    in Phase I dinner, 48, 51–52
    in Phase I lunch, 37–38
    root, as green-light food, 68
vegetarian omelet, 75
vegetarians, 50
vinaigrette, basic, 78
vitamins, 122–23
    RDA of, 121

W
waist circumference, 17
    weekly log for, 152

Waldorf chicken and rice salad, 80
walking, 108–9, 110–11
Wall Street Journal, 4
warm-ups, 143
water, in Phase I, 52–53
weight, weight loss:
    BMI and, 16–17, *18–19*
    cardiovascular disease and, 118–19
    diabetes, 119–20
    exercise and, 108–10
    fad diets and, xi–xii
    and maintenance, 108–10
    pound-per-week goal in, 22
    timetable for, *23*
    weekly log for, 152
Western omelet, 75
wheat, processing of, 7–8
wheat bran, *see* bran
white flour, 7
wine, 99, 101
Wine Spectator, 99
wraps, 40–41
W exercises, 148

Y
yellow-light foods, 22–23, 125–32
    in Phase I breakfast, 30–32
    in Phase I dinner, 46–49
    in Phase I lunch, 36–39
    in Phase I snacks, 45
yogurt, yogurt cheese, as green-light
    food, 69, 91

Z
Zone, The (Sears), xiii
Zone Diet, xiii
    early complexity of, xiv–xv
    G.I. diet versus, xv